Improve Your Vision

Also by Martin Brofman

Anything Can Be Healed
244-page paperback, ISBN 1-84409-016-7

White Light Vision Improvement
CD, ISBN 1-84409-026-4

Healing Vibrations
CD, ISBN 1-84409-024-8

Stay in the White Light, & Dream
CD, ISBN 1-84409-023-X

You Know You Are a Healer
CD, ISBN 1-84409-025-6

all published by FINDHORN PRESS
available from your local bookstore
or directly from www.findhornpress.com

Improve Your Vision

Your Inner Guide to Clearer Vision

Martin Brofman

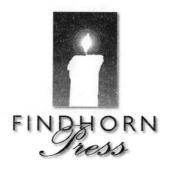

FINDHORN
Press

© Martin Brofman 2004
First published by Findhorn Press in 2004

ISBN 1-84409-030-2

British Library Cataloguing-in-Publication Data.
A catalogue record for this book is available from the British Library.

Edited by Elaine Harrison
Cover and interior design by Thierry Bogliolo
Cover photograph © DigitalVision

Printed and bound by WS Bookwell, Finland

Published by

Findhorn Press
305a The Park, Findhorn
Forres IV36 3TE
Scotland
Tel 01309 690582
Fax 01309 690036
e-mail: info@findhornpress.com
www.findhornpress.com

Contents

Preface

Dr. Bates was the first to propose the idea that eyesight could be corrected. Since the official position of the optometric community was (and in many places still is) that eyesight couldn't be corrected, his ideas were considered very controversial. Throughout the controversy, however, there remained one inescapable fact – in some cases vision actually improved! How could there be any argument with success? Some of his successes included such disorders as glaucoma, cataracts, and retinitis pigmentosa.

One of Dr. Bates' basic premises was that all impaired vision is always accompanied by a particular mental state. Further research by Charles Kelley of the Radix Institute showed how particular mental states accompany each particular kind of impaired vision. My experience is that a person's vision is indeed a metaphor for their state of consciousness, that a person's way of Being is directly related to their way of seeing.

The long-standing idea had been that the eye functions like a box camera, with the accommodation process accomplished by functions within the eye, such as the action of the ciliary muscles varying the thickness of the lens. This was known as the Helmholtz Theory. Dr. Bates, however, proposed that the eye functions more like a bellows camera. He suggested the extrinsic muscles surrounding it controlled the variable length of the eyeball, and that tension in these eye muscles could be released, resulting in clearer vision. He also implied tension in these muscles was related to particular mental tension – supporting the metaphoric significance of impaired vision at the level of consciousness.

Dr. Bates found that not only were people with eye problems mentally tense in some way; they were also physically tense in their bodies. Consequently, many of his techniques were geared to creating a mental state of relaxation through imagining calming scenes and physical relaxation techniques.

Margaret Darst Corbett, who was trained by Dr. Bates, and also worked with Aldous Huxley, carried on Dr. Bates' work after his death in 1931. Mrs. Corbett noted that faulty eyesight seemed always to be accompanied by faulty breathing – another aspect of body tension – and noticed that when her students were encouraged to breathe easily, their eyesight improved.

Having studied the ideas of Wilhelm Reich and Alexander Lowen, Dr. Kelley felt that the true cause of visual disorders is in the person's inability to express deep feelings.

Each of the approaches mentioned is related in some way to the others, and all of them have proven useful to some degree.

The question in many minds has been, "So why haven't these processes been more successful?" For even though many successes have been reported, there have also been many people who have diligently applied themselves, and had only limited success.

It is the opinion of this author that success only comes with willingness on a person's part to make the necessary changes in their consciousness, in their way of Being, in the way they make their life work for themselves. All of the successes I have seen have been accompanied by dramatic changes in the person's lifestyle; changes of such magnitude that the improvement in vision was considered by many to be a side benefit of the process they had gone through. In my own case, normal vision returned without working on it at all, but rather focusing on what I needed to do in order to be happy. After all, a happy person experiences less stress than an unhappy person, and stress affects vision adversely.

Bates' approach has been considered by many to be too technical and mechanical. Although the ideas in his book show a deep insight into the processes of consciousness that accompany impaired vision, many of those using his techniques overlook these ideas and focus instead on the outer form of what they are doing, rather than their inner experience while doing it. Consequently, their success is then limited.

In one case I have known, a man was able to reduce his prescription from 16 diopters to 12 diopters in three months by just using physical relaxation techniques, but he was not willing to explore the deeper dimensions of his impaired vision, so there was no further improvement. Even so – he was able to see a bird for the first time in his life!

In this book, the primary emphasis is on the internal process, that which goes on in your consciousness. This is a process of deep personal transformation. The techniques are, by and large, mental techniques. *Improve Your Vision* can provide the motivation, inspiration, and tools for the transformation process, offering you the opportunity to change both your way of Being and your way of seeing. It is you, the reader, who must use the tools in order for them to work.

There may be some apprehension experienced, since we all tend to justify our way of Being, and many are hesitant to change and maybe 'become someone else'. What actually happens is you become more yourself – who you really are. You peel the layers off and rediscover your true self.

If you have impaired vision, you have not been yourself; you have hidden or suppressed your real self, or lived according to an image of what you think you 'should' be. Can you imagine what your life will be like when you discover you don't have to do that, and you can be the real YOU? Will you feel freer?

This book can be your vehicle to the life you've always wanted, in which you are happy, relaxed, and see clearly. When you are happy and relaxed you experience less stress and tension. When stress and tension leave your consciousness, they also leave your body, along with any impaired vision symptoms, and you return to balance on all levels.

Can this book teach you how to be happy? No. You already know how to do that. All it takes is for you to do what makes you happy, and stop doing what makes you unhappy. However, you have been keeping yourself from happiness – even from seeing what it is that would make you happy – and doubting you can really have it. This book can remind you of the things that, deep inside, you've always known were true.

Are you now willing to see?

Are you willing to make the changes to transform?

Can this book help you do that?

Yes it can.

Disclaimer:

Healing and Medicine are two very different disciplines and the law requires the following disclaimer. The information in this book is not medicine but healing and does not constitute medical advice. In case of serious illness consult the practitioner of your choice.

Introduction

This is a book about Vision Improvement, but it much more than a book about eyesight; it is about finding inner clarity. Clarity within will lead to clear vision. I can state this because I have experienced it, and have witnessed many more do just the same. My own journey to clarity began with a huge 'wake-up call' and I would like to share my story with you by way of an introduction to what follows.

I had terminal cancer in 1975 and was told that I had just one or two months to live. The tumor was in my spinal cord – in the neck – and as it grew it was pressing the spinal cord against the inside of the spinal canal. My right arm had become paralyzed, and my legs were spastic. An operation to remove the tumor had been unsuccessful, and I was told that for various reasons chemotherapy and radiation therapy would not work.

Doctors warned me the end might come very suddenly, any moment, if I coughed or sneezed. I was faced with a reality in which each day was possibly my last day, each hour my last hour. One thing I knew for sure – for whatever time I had remaining, I wanted to be happy, just being myself. For that reason, unappealing special diets made no sense to me, despite the claims they may help. Each meal was possibly my last meal and I wanted to eat what I really enjoyed. I had to be true to myself, to be real in all that I did.

My values shifted. I lived in the present moment and everything I did was for its own sake, because I really wanted to do it. Some things that had seemed important before suddenly weren't any more. The only important thing was being happy and to me that meant doing whatever I felt happy doing, and not doing anything that made me unhappy.

Two months later, I was still alive; I had run out of time, but I was still alive! One month later I was on overtime, and *still* alive. I wondered how long it could go on. New Year was five months away and I decided that if by some miracle I was still here, I would celebrate with a vacation in a tropical paradise. What I didn't know then was how that vacation would save my life.

Five months later, I was celebrating the New Year in Martinique, having a mind-expanding talk with a man who was there to teach Zen meditation. He said to me:

"Cancer begins in your mind, and that's where you can go to get rid of it".

It was like someone had switched a light bulb on – it was so clear. I knew what he meant and could see how the cancer was a metaphor for things held in and not expressed. I saw how my former lifestyle and way of being had led to me killing myself in many ways. I realized there and then that if I changed my way of being, I could somehow release the symptoms. I could use my mind as a tool to accomplish the changes in my way of being, and in my body.

For the first time since I had been given the diagnosis, I was able to consider a possibility of turning around my condition and getting rid of the cancer. I could save my life!

Several weeks later, I listened to a talk about Silva Mind Control (now renamed the Silva Method), which teaches people how to use their mind as a tool. The idea presented was that our perceptions create our reality, and since we choose our perceptions, we can choose to change any aspect of our reality. My consciousness had been the effect of programming; in the same way that a computer produces results based on how it has been programmed. *I* could reprogram *my* consciousness.

My perception had been that *I was terminally ill,* so I had to reprogram my consciousness to create the perception that *I was well.* I was not prepared for such an abrupt shift. For some considerable time I had perceived myself as being in a state of deterioration, getting closer and closer to dying. This called for a major change in my thinking. I realized that I could much more easily create the perception that *I was getting better and better*, until *I was* eventually *well*.

I knew the turnaround could happen in any moment. It was a matter of turning a switch in my mind, and insisting on knowing it had been turned. I decided that if the moment of change could be any moment, then let it be *now*.

The shift in my consciousness was immediate, I felt it, and I knew then that I was in a state of improvement. I also knew the importance of maintaining the integrity of my decision. From that moment on I knew that my perceptions had to reinforce the idea I was now getting better and better, so I would eventually be well.

As I ate whatever food I wanted, I told myself it was exactly what my body needed and was asking for in order to accelerate the healing process. Physical sensations similar to electric shocks in my body had previously reinforced the idea that the tumor was growing. They still came, but now I chose to perceive them as evidence that the tumor was shrinking.

My mind looked for more and more ways of knowing the improvement was happening.

I knew I had to stay away from people who insisted on seeing me as still terminally ill, not from any lack of love, but rather to maintain my own positive attitude toward the healing process. I had to be with people who were willing to encourage me on this seemingly impossible task I had set for myself. Whenever someone asked how I was doing, I insisted on answering, "Better and Better, thank-you". And it was true.

I researched mental programming techniques, and learnt that if I put myself into a relaxed state and talked positively to myself for 15 minutes, three times a day, then within 66 days I could get myself to believe anything. And whatever I believed to be true would be true.

I knew that it was vital to maintain the positive programming, and that putting myself in a relaxed state of mind and talking positively to myself for 15 minutes, three times each day, was a part of the programming process I should in no way interfere with. There were temptations to not do the relaxations, and then I would remind myself that my life was at stake. Any such temptation, then, was something that stood between me and my life, and had to be removed, so that I could live.

This may all sound very simple, but it was not always easy. At times – especially early on – it was very difficult. Sometimes my thoughts or words acknowledged something other than the idea that I was improving. On such occasions I had to be honest with myself and see that I had 'blown it'. I would start again, telling myself I had been on a practice run, and the real moment of change was *now*.

It did get easier. I was able to maintain positivity and integrity for just hours at first, then a day, then two days, and then I was solid. The program was working.

The doubting voice would occasionally make itself known, but I knew it did not represent truth. The encouraging voice within became my guide, leading me back to stable health, enabling me to maintain the single-mindedness of knowing positive changes were happening. When I was not feeling a symptom, I told myself that perhaps I would never feel that symptom again. If I did then experience the symptom again I would tell myself the process was not quite complete, but to acknowledge I was feeling the symptom less often and less severely than before. All was going well.

I had to know positive changes were happening now even if they were not always evident. I would tell myself they were possibly just at the threshold of my perception, so I could eagerly anticipate evidence to justify this. I was always able to find something positive, and assure myself it wasn't all imagination.

There was much encouragement from my daughters, Jacki and Heather. Heather was only four years old at the time and she knew that love heals, so she gave me magic healing kisses – every morning and every night. I could also sense six-year-old Jacki's belief in me, and in my ability to somehow come through this crisis. No other possibility was acceptable to her. In her eyes, I could always see her connection with me.

During my relaxation periods, I would visualize the tumor and imagine a layer of cancer cells dying and being released by my body's natural elimination system. I knew the change was happening, even if it was not obvious and noticeable. Each time I released waste products from my body I knew dead cancer cells were being eliminated. I insisted on knowing this was true.

I knew the cancer represented something held in and not expressed. With the tumor located right by my throat chakra (energy center) I also knew this meant I had been holding back the expression of my Being. Since I wasn't exactly certain what this meant I decided it was imperative to express everything: every thought and every feeling. Whatever was in my consciousness and wanting to come out, I expressed it, knowing it was vital for my health. Before then I had held the perception that expressing led to discord, but now I saw how what I was expressing and communicating was appreciated by those around me and resulted in harmony.

Before, I had had the belief that if I expressed what I really wanted to, something bad would happen. I had to reprogram that to the belief that if I expressed what I really wanted to, something wonderful would happen. I made that decision, and it was so.

I found myself having less and less in common with my old friends. It was as though we had shared a common vibrational frequency before, say 547 cycles (whatever that means), and suddenly I found myself at 872 cycles, with few things to communicate to the 547-cycle people. I had to find new friends who were also at 872 so I could have someone to talk with.

I found myself attracted to the 872 crowd, and them to me, as though I had become selectively magnetic. Certain elements of my reality were being released which were no longer in accord with the new Being I was becoming. Deep within I knew the process was inevitable and should not be interfered with. I developed a sense of compassion and understanding and knew my life depended on releasing all elements not in accord with my new vibration. The process was simple, though not always easy.

I began each day as a process of self-discovery, with no preconceived notion of who I was, but with a willingness to discover the emerging me. There was a sense of delight with each new discovery.

Often I would imagine the scene in the doctor's office after my work on myself was done. I would see him examining me and looking puzzled because he could find no tumor. I imagined him looking baffled and saying, "Perhaps we made a mistake." I played this scene in my mind each day, during my relaxation periods.

About two months later I went to be examined by the very same doctor who had pronounced me terminally ill. He examined me and he found nothing. And guess what he said? "Perhaps we made a mistake." I laughed all the way home.

I have transformed my way of Being. My lifestyle has changed dramatically. I had been working on Wall Street, designing computer systems and involved in computer fraud. While it was interesting, I didn't feel it so important in the 'bigger picture'. I was commuting 90 minutes each way to and from work, and living 'the American Dream' – a house in the suburbs, a wife and two children, two cars in the garage, a big dog… but I wasn't happy.

Working with consciousness, it feels as though I have moved up to a higher class of computer. The work I do now as a healer and teacher is meaningful to me, important to others, and of service to humanity. I feel a 'high' when I heal and teach and I know that I am doing my life's work.

The process of transformation is an integral part of the healing process, whether you're healing your vision, releasing some serious illness, or if the imbalance exists on the mental or emotional level and has not yet reached the physical level.

An unexpected but wonderful side benefit of my healing process was that I no longer needed the eyeglasses I had worn for twenty years. I used to be nearsighted and astigmatic, but my vision changed and my eyesight was tested as 'normal'.

After my healing I was seeing the world quite differently, in a figurative and a literal sense. My outer vision had been transformed along with my inner vision. Curious about this 'side benefit' of my healing process I decided to research into what others were doing in the field of vision improvement.

I read all the books I could find on the subject, not because I needed to find out 'how to do it', but rather to discover 'how I had done it'. I found eight books, and seven of them referred back to the eighth, which was *Better Eyesight Without Glasses*, by Dr. William Bates. He was a pioneer in the field, and his ideas had startled the conventional medical community back in the 1920's.

Dr. Bates presented many remarkable ideas, but the style of his book was way too technical for many people, so others – like Margaret Darst Corbett and Aldous Huxley – wrote additional books, simplifying his ideas for the general public.

Dr. Charles Kelley of the Radix Institute in California was the first one who seemed to add new ideas, regarding the correlation of particular personality types to particular types of impaired vision. More recently, Dr. Richard Kavner, a behavioral optometrist, added some new information regarding brain/mind correlations and he achieved remarkable success through his work with children.

The constant factor in all these areas of vision improvement was the process of personal transformation – just as in my own personal experience. With the insight I gained by reading the works of those mentioned, I was able to build on their ideas, using my personal experience for additional insights.

I began talking to people about these ideas and helping them to explore the links between their own vision issues and their way of being. After a while, those I spoke to were giving me their eyeglass-es, saying they no longer needed them.

Since 1975, I have worked with tens of thousands of people, watching many of them improve their eyesight by retraining their consciousness, and changing their lives in the process. In fact, the magnitude of change in their lives has often been such that these people consider their improved eyesight a relatively minor aspect of the whole.

This book is the result of the research I have done, and the experiences I have had functioning as a guide for those people who have transformed their vision. Rather than the 'outer' processes (diet, physical movements, exercise, vitamins, etc.), which are often focused on by many other approaches to vision improvement, this book mainly focuses on the 'inner' processes. This is a book about what happens in our consciousness, the place from where everything in our experience begins. As we release tensions in our consciousness and accept new ideas, tensions are also released from the physical body and we return to balance on all levels.

Dr. Bates stated that all impaired vision was the result of stress. When we think of impaired vision, we think not only of the organic mechanics of vision, but also about the function of vision, about what you experience visually. According to Dr. Bates, if we forget about the mechanics of vision and concentrate only on the function of vision – the experience in our consciousness – then when the function of vision is restored, the organic 'causes' of impaired vision are also reversed.

The orientation of this book is for errors of refraction (nearsightedness, farsightedness, and astigmatism). However, people who have had what are known as 'organic' visual difficulties (cataracts, glaucoma, etc.) have also reported improvement after conscientiously applying the ideas contained herein, as well as other self-healing concepts. These include the idea that they were totally responsible for their condition, that it was the result of particular perceptions they chose to have, and therefore that they were able to change it, by changing their attitudes.

May you, the reader, find the contents of this book useful and valuable. My wish is that it can aid your return to a state of Being where you are able to totally experience your wholeness, and your natural state of clarity.

How to Use This Book

First, read the book through and get a sense of the process described. At the end of the book, you will find a recommended two-month program, with three levels of involvement: good, excellent, and optimal.

Decide which level of involvement you are comfortable with and be certain it's a program to which you can commit yourself. It's often better to choose a lighter level, which you can easily do, rather than a deeper level you will not be able to maintain. Whatever level you choose, commit to doing it. Make it a part of your daily regimen – a high priority project – and do it regardless of any conditions that present themselves. After all it is important – it's your eyesight...and much more besides!

Build a pattern of success with the program. The deeper you get into it, the more results you will see.

I recommend that after reading the book through once, you then re-read one chapter each day. There are many different levels of information contained herein. The same words will make sense in a different way when you re-read them, plus your experiences will begin to relate to what you are reading.

As you read the descriptions appropriate to the type of impaired vision you experience, look for the way the words describe you, and recognize the way of Being you have experienced that has been related to your way of seeing.

At the end of each chapter there are affirmations which are in some way related to its contents. During your day, think of those affirmations, and what they mean to you. Repeat the affirmations to yourself as often as you can during the day – perhaps once each hour or two. These affirmations will help to re-orient your consciousness, returning you once more to your natural state of clarity.

There may be times when your progress is rapid, and other times when it seems slower and more difficult, but keep at it. In the grand scale of things, two months of your life is not such a long time, and it will be time well spent. Be willing to look at all of those issues you have been avoiding looking at, and see what it will take for you to be happy.

Trust the process.

It works.

You will see.

Section 1

Being and Seeing

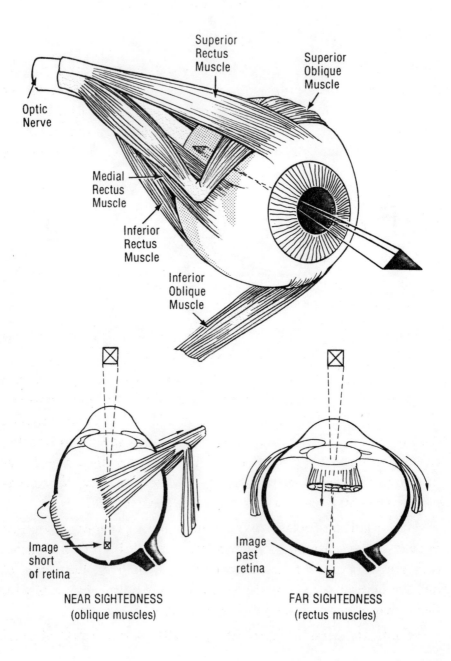

Superior
Rectus
Muscle

Superior
Oblique
Muscle

Optic
Nerve

Medial
Rectus
Muscle

Inferior
Rectus
Muscle

Inferior
Oblique
Muscle

Image
short
of retina

Image
past
retina

NEAR SIGHTEDNESS
(oblique muscles)

FAR SIGHTEDNESS
(rectus muscles)

Chapter 1

Vision as a Metaphor

Look into someone's eyes and you will see who they really are. We may be able to force smiles and say what others want to hear, but the truth is always right there in our eyes. Eyes cannot lie. Our physical eyes are the organs of outer perception, but they also relate to our inner perceptions. Our language is sprinkled liberally with references to the metaphor of vision:

> *"He's SO short sighted"*
> *"She is such a visionary"*
> *"He refuses to see what is happening!"*
> *"I see"*
> *"They are blind to his ways"*
> *"He refuses to look at the issue"*

and so on – yet none of these are about physical eyesight. So what is this relationship between our eyesight and our way of Being?

Eyesight is not just a physical process involving acuity; it is a multi-dimensional function affecting and affected by our emotional and mental state of Being. Eyesight is also linked to personality and each type of vision impairment correlates with a specific personality type. *(Please note: If you skipped this book's introduction, then I urge you at this stage to go back and read it – you will find a very clear example of how outer vision is a reflection of an inner process.)*

Nearsighted people all have something in common, farsighted people share a particular character trait, and all those with astigmatism are working with a similar issue in their lives. Each type of impaired vision represents the stressed way a person interacts with their environment, a way that is not 'at ease'.

Some say stress is responsible for all emotional and physical imbalances – it certainly accounts for a vast amount of time off work and doctors recognize its role in the creation of illness (or dis-ease). Stress is stored in the physical body in a number of ways, including tightness or tension in particular muscles. Stress headaches and tense shoulders are two common examples.

We can say, then, that physical tension is emotional or mental tension stored in the muscles of the physical body. Tension in specific muscles is related to particular emotions and mental states. In other words, *where* you feel the tension is related to *why* you feel the tension. In the case of vision, different visual disorders have been linked with excessive tension in particular extra-ocular muscles (the muscles surrounding the eyeballs), and with particular emotional patterns.

Surrounding each eyeball are six eye muscles (see illustration on page 22). We use these muscles to move our eyeballs in different directions, and for a while it was thought this was their only function. However, it was then discovered these muscles are about one hundred times more powerful than they need to be to accomplish this movement. Since structure and function are related in the human body, it seemed evident these muscles must have another function. They do.

The extra-ocular muscles also serve as part of the focusing mechanism for our eyesight, along with the lens. They cause the eyeballs to elongate or shorten depending on what we are looking at, and what we are thinking or feeling. In this way, the eye operates like a bellows camera, with variable focus – as opposed to a box camera with a fixed focal length.

Four Rectus muscles pull each eyeball straight back into the eye socket, shortening the eyeball. Excessive tension on these muscles creates a condition of farsightedness. This tension is also experienced emotionally, as a background feeling of anger, or as guilt (anger at one's Self). It can be experienced as a sense of coming out of one's Self and focusing on an external image or role rather than who one truly is. In the farsighted person, energy is expanding and holding –

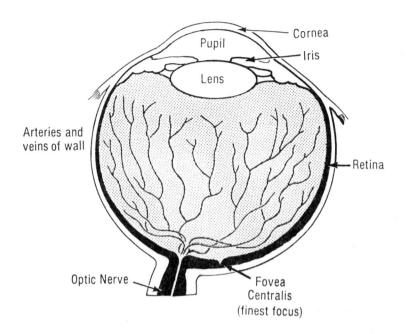

Cornea

Pupil

Iris

Lens

Arteries and
veins of wall

Retina

Optic Nerve

Fovea
Centralis
(finest focus)

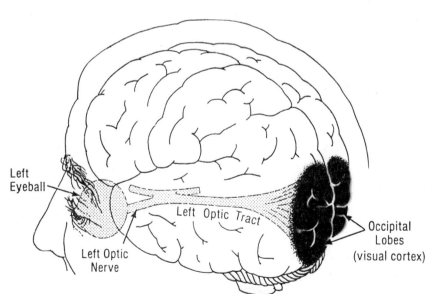

Left
Eyeball

Left Optic Tract

Left Optic
Nerve

Occipital
Lobes
(visual cortex)

even pushing – things away. There can be a feeling that in some way the individual is not as important as others.

Two muscles circle around each eyeball like a belt, these are called the Oblique muscles. When these muscles are tightened, they squeeze the eyeball, causing it to elongate. Excessive tension on these muscles is related to nearsightedness and this tension is experienced emotionally as hiding within one's Self, retreating inward. This may be experienced as apprehension, fear, mistrust, a sense of feeling threatened, or not feeling safe to be one's Self. It may be experienced as all of these.

Uneven tensions on different muscles squeeze the eyeball unevenly, pulling the eyeball out of roundness and creating a condition of astigmatism – a distortion of vision. This can be experienced by the individual as a sense of being lost, of being uncertain or confused about their values – about what they really want or what they really feel. Values from the 'outside' have been included 'inside', in a way that is not natural or real for the individual. The stress of this situation is experienced in the person's consciousness as well as in the eye muscles.

Impaired vision comes about in people's lives when they are experiencing stress in relation to their environment, when they are not seeing clearly – both literally and figuratively. If this goes on for an extended period of time, the eye muscles holding these tensions can become temporarily 'frozen', holding the eyeball in an out-of-focus condition. Since the tensions in these muscles correspond with tensions in the person's consciousness, this also holds the individual in a particular state of consciousness. The good news is these eye muscles can be relaxed and clear vision restored using relaxation techniques and Hatha Yoga eye exercises (similar to what optometrists call motility training).

When the proper tone is restored to the eye muscles, the eyeballs are able to resume their natural shape and clear vision can return. Tensions are also released in the person's body and consciousness, resulting in a return to an easier, clearer, more natural way of Being.

The natural state of our vision is clear, and a return to clarity is a return to our natural state of balance and really being ourselves.

We can also return to clarity and balance by addressing the way we live our lives, rather than focusing on our eye muscles. Vision is a metaphor for the way we see the world and is related to personality. Once the elements of a person's experience that relate to their impaired vision are identified and released, then clear vision can be restored. By releasing the excessive tensions in our consciousness we can release tensions from the eye muscles and our eyeballs can return to their natural shape, resulting in clear vision.

Since each type of vision impairment corresponds to a particular personality type, a change in personality can be expected alongside a change in outer vision. The 'new' will have the same essence of Being as the 'old', but will enjoy a different way of interacting with the environment – a different dance.

Such a change is like having a perceptual filter removed – a filter through which values had previously been determined. Rather than being at the effect of perceptions we know to be distortions, we can decide to be at the cause. We can decide to consciously align with and choose those perceptions we know to be really true for us, and which will be more successful for us in our interactions, more in keeping with who we really are. Without the old filter, new values become evident and the consequences can be far reaching. Changes can be as simple as new and different tastes in food, clothing and music – a consequence of being true to yourself for a change. Or they can be as major as career and relationship changes. Such changes may sound radical, but they will always be for the best, ultimately leading to greater happiness and fulfillment.

Approaches to vision improvement which have not considered the aspect of personality change have had only limited success. In cases where vision has been restored, the person involved has been through a transformative process and has, in fact, dropped a role. They have become another Being, with another personality, more real, and with another way of seeing the world. The degree of improvement and the rapidity of improvement has been connected with the willingness on the part of the individual to accept the changes, to accept the new personality, to become the new Being, or rather, to become and live who they really are.

If we imagine that each of us is surrounded by a bubble of energy, our individual perceptual filters, we can see some metaphors.

Nearsightedness

People who are nearsighted see what is close to them easier than they see what is far away. They are more focused on what is inside their bubble, and less on what is outside. Energy – the direction of attention – is toward the inside, and away from the outside, moving inward and contracting, and things must be close in order to be seen clearly and comfortably. One's orientation is toward Self, to an excess for that person, where 'I' is considered more important than 'you', and 'we' does not seem to include 'you' as an equal consideration. What they want or feel is experienced as more important to them than what others want or feel. Nearsighted people often have an exceptional need for privacy and can be withdrawn from the world around them. They may feel intimidated by their environment, and have a sense of hiding inside.

For nearsighted people, the focus of thinking is forward, with fear or uncertainty as the emotional experience of that view. This preoccupation with the future keeps the individual from being totally present – in the here and now – and the degree to which this is experienced is related to the degree of nearsightedness. There may also be different compensations in the personality, such as aggression to mask and minimize the intimidation, or a forced extraversion to disguise the hiding within, but what we are talking about here is the inner basis behind these outer actions.

Farsightedness

People who are farsighted see what is further away more easily than what is close to them. Farsighted people are more focused on what is outside their bubble and less on what is inside. Energy – the direction of attention – is expanding and moving outward, holding away of moving against what is outside. Things must be held at a distance to be seen clearly and comfortably. What others want or feel is experienced as more important than the individual's own wants or feelings and there is an excessive orientation toward others and away from Self. 'You' is considered more important than 'I', and 'we' does not seem to include 'I' as an equal consideration.

While a nearsighted person retreats witin readily and easily, a farsighted person has difficulty doing this, since their attention continues to be directed outward. A farsighted person is interested in other people's lives and avoids looking at their own. Their image (how they appear to others) is over-emphasized and identified with, gaining more importance to them than their essence – who they *really* are. Any sense of anger may be suppressed, so as not to offend others. The focus of thinking is in the past, often with anger and self-justification, or a sense of not having done the 'right thing'. This preoccupation with the past keeps the individual from being totally present. Again, the degree to which this is true is a matter of individual balance, and the degree of farsightedness experienced by the individual. There may be outer compensatory behavior, such as exaggerated saintliness to hide the guilt, or extreme kindliness to cover the anger.

Astigmatism

People with astigmatism experience uncertainty of wants

or feelings, depending on whether the right, the left, or both eyes is affected. Their 'bubble' is distorted.

Metaphysically, the right eye (the Will eye) represents clearly seeing what one wants, and the left eye (the Spirit eye) represents clearly seeing what one feels (in left-handed people, the traits are reversed). A person with astigmatism wants or feels what is true for them, considers it inappropriate and then changes it. They then believe the pretended change, no longer seeing clearly what they really wanted or felt in the first instance. The focus is more on what 'should' be wanted or felt, rather than what is real for them. A sense of confusion results about who they really are. Who would they be if they stopped pretending to be who they are not?

Combinations of visual disorders are related to combinations of the qualities already mentioned. Astigmatism may be experienced in combination with either nearsightedness or farsightedness. Of course the personality traits mentioned may also be experienced without the visual disorders, but for individuals with impaired vision these traits are particularly strong.

Nearsightedness means seeing more clearly up close. Farsightedness means seeing more clearly far away. While in some rare cases one eye may be nearsighted and the other farsighted, both conditions may not exist within the same eye. When a person sees neither near nor far with clarity, the condition is one of rigidity of the accommodation mechanism, reflecting rigidity of consciousness. Relaxation techniques and eye exercises can restore flexibility. As a result, the individual will also notice greater flexibility in their mental process.

We are Beings of energy, and energy is directed by our consciousness. Ultimately, we have the capability of choosing the direction of the flow of energy in any situation. We can choose to not be directed by past patterns. We can change those perceptions we know to be less than accurate or optimal, and be willing to see things as they really are, rather than through a distorting filter.

The flow of energy between the inside and the outside of the bubble can be changed, as can the nature of the bubble itself. Remember, this is the perceptual 'filter' through which we perceive our environment. A 'stuck' filter predisposes us to particular patterns of interacting and perceiving. It's like a selective lens, only allowing through perceptions that agree with the basic beliefs we have chosen or accepted, while ignoring or discounting all others. Since we act on the basis of the information that gets through to us, we are then predisposed to responding to our environment in a fixed way. The selectivity of the lens is not the problem, though – the distorting quality of the emotional filter is what must be released.

When we are clear and centered, the bubble is clear and so are our interactions. When we are in the middle of a strong emotion, we are not centered and the bubble is not clear, as it is distorted with the emotional currents. When these emotional currents distort the bubble, situations look different and we respond differently. We can often recognize that our view had been distorted, sometimes even during the moment of experience. When the strong emotions of anger, fear, confusion, etc., are *suppressed*, as is the case with those who have impaired vision, the bubble is also distorted, but the distortion is not recognized. The person identifies with the distorted view and believes that it represents truth, and who they really are. In fact, it is not who they are, but just who they seem to be when functioning with the distortion. They can release the distorting aspect of the lens, and of their perceptions, and return to their true clear selves.

Making changes – From Near to Clear

Nearsighted people can direct the energy outward by being more and more willing to be visible and trust they will be safe doing so, letting people see who they really are. They can learn to see themselves through other people's eyes, understanding how others see them, so they not only have the view from the inside looking out, but also from the outside looking in. This will give them the opportunity to step outside themselves and see things from another point of view and with the additional information thus gained, to use it to optimize their interactions.

It is also important to treat the other person as they themselves would like to be treated if they were in the other person's place. It isn't necessary to agree with the other person's perceptions of them, but just have the willingness to see that's how they are being seen, and that the other person's perceptions are as important to the other person as their own are to them. In fact, the other person's perceptions might be very useful to know about.

Nearsighted people benefit from working on their self-confidence, and choosing to no longer make decisions based on fear. The idea is to not feel threatened or intimidated by the environment in which the individuals find themselves, but rather to focus more and more on letting themselves be themselves, letting themselves be real. It's about trusting that when they do what they *really want to do*, then something wonderful always happens. And since this process is so important for our-*selves*, nearsighted people must also learn to recognize how the same process is important for other people, too, and that everyone is just getting better and better at being themselves.

Making changes – From Far to Clear

Farsighted people can redirect the energy inward by giving themselves the same consideration they give others. The idea is not to stop considering others, but to also consider their own self in the same way – to do for themselves what they are ready to do for others. This can involve a conscious process of allowing themselves to receive without guilt – not to take, but to receive, to accept (notice the difference). It is also important for them to express wants and feelings – to let themselves have. When receiving, there is no need to reciprocate or deny, but just say, "Thank you" and accept unconditionally. This acceptance can apply to ideas, too, and they should notice ways they have been holding things, ideas, or even people away. The focus can be switched to who they really are, rather than their image. Image is important, but Essence must not be overlooked. Outer appearance is not more important than true sentiment, and people do appreciate honesty in feelings.

Consideration must also extend to yourself. Expressing love need not involve sacrifice. It's not necessary to come out of your space to be loved and respected. The role can be fun, but also remember the Being who is playing it, the person inside. From the farsighted person's point of view, 'WE' can include 'I' as equal to 'YOU,' and 'I' can be seen as another 'YOU,' as well as separate and important in its own right.

Making changes – Astigmatism

Astigmatics can ask themselves from time to time, during their day, "What do I really want now? What do I really feel now? What's true for me? What's real for me? If I stop wanting to be what I'm not, who would I be? If I stop living up to other people's standards, who would I be?" If I stop pretending to be the person I've been playing, what would I be doing differently?

The feeling may have been that who the person really is would not be accepted in the environment in which the individual finds himself or herself. The idea, then, is to find out whether the feeling is real, by discontinuing the role, and just being themselves. They will either discover the feeling was a misperception and the role was unnecessary, or that the feeling was real, in which case they would have the option of migrating to another environment in which they can be themselves, and be accepted. Either way, the effect will be a greater sense of ease in being who they really are.

There's a place in society for all of us. If we let ourselves be real, there's a place where we all fit in, where we are accepted and appreciated for who we are. We do not have to pretend not to see what's real for us. We can all allow ourselves to be who we really are, to be more and more real.

With determination and a willingness to change perceptions and their accompanying realities, anyone can transform their view of the world – both literally and figuratively – and return to a natural state of clarity of vision.

Affirmations

It's more and more comfortable to be myself and to see clearly.

I know I can see clearly without eyeglasses.

As I clear my life, my vision clears.

Chapter 2

Returning to Clarity

If you have made the decision to transform your vision, several things should be considered.

You must deeply want the change to happen, and you must be willing to do what is necessary – in a sense, to make it a high priority project, perhaps the most important thing in your life, at least for a time. Two months is a reasonable time to devote to your vision. During that time, it's helpful if there is an established routine. A recommended two-month program is found at the end of this book. There should be a willingness to dedicate yourself for the two months, and at the end of that time, to see the degree of improvement that is noticeable and measurable.

During the transformation period, insist on knowing your vision and eyesight are improving. Any doubting voice inside must be disregarded, and your encouraging voice must be identified with. Know deep within yourself that the changes are happening, regardless of any so-called 'evidence' to the contrary.

The fact of the ongoing improvement must be a 'given' in your consciousness. If blurriness is experienced, know it is not because the process isn't working; it is because the process is not yet complete. If clarity has not yet been experienced, then know it is still in the process of happening.

Always encourage the perception that changes are happening now, possibly just at the threshold of notice-ability. Anticipate the changes eagerly and watch for evidence they are actually happening *right* now. Notice how you can see clearer than you used to – even if it feels like it might just be your imagination! You will soon know that it is not something you are just imagining, but real, and the personal re-assurance will give additional strength to the process.

Stress and tension are the causes of impaired vision and concern about eyesight increases stress, so it can become a self-fulfilling prophecy. In a sense, it is helpful if you are not emotionally involved in the process. Become the observer and patiently and optimistically watch for the changes to become evident. If you feel stressed about the non-clarity of your vision, the stress in your consciousness will go into the extra-ocular muscles, making them squeeze harder and hold the eyeball even more out of shape.

Meet your vision where it is at right now – let it be what it is. Like watching a movie on soft focus, if you don't see the details too well, then enjoy the colors, or the shapes and movements instead. As you relax, stress is released from your consciousness and your eye muscles, and consequently your vision will clear. It's a bit like watching a television set fine-tuning itself with no effort on your part. You just watch it happen.

It is helpful if you only wear your eyeglasses when absolutely necessary – for instance, if doing an activity would be impossible or unsafe without the glasses. Driving a car, for example, may require eyeglasses, whereas talking to people or listening to music does not. When the glasses are not necessary to the function being performed, remove them and free your consciousness from dependency on them.

When your eyes were examined, you had certain tensions in your consciousness, which were reflected in the tensions in your eye muscles. These tensions held your eyeball in a particular shape and created a particular experience of vision specific to that time. The lenses you were given compensated for your vision in that moment. When the lenses were placed in front of your eyes, they compensated for your vision as experienced with that shape of eyeball, with those particular tensions in your eye muscles and in your consciousness.

Several days later, when you put on the new glasses, you felt uncomfortable with them, and were told that your eyes had to get adjusted to the lenses. Why should that be, when they had just adjusted the lenses to your eyes?

What makes more sense is that several days later, after your eye examination, there were different tensions in your consciousness, creating different tensions in your eye muscles, and a different shape to your eyeball, different from what it was at the time that your eyes were examined. Now, in order to see clearly through the lenses, you had to create the same eyeball shape you had on the day you were tested, by creating the same tensions in your eye muscles, by creating the same tensions in your consciousness.

Just as your eyeglasses have held your eyes in a fixed focus, they have held your consciousness in a fixed focus, too. They have held your consciousness in the state it was in when your eyes were examined – at a time in your life when you were experiencing a great deal of stress (otherwise you would have not needed the eyeglasses!).

You have worn these tensions, then, in your consciousness. You have become accustomed to them, and identified with them as being who you are, even though you are no longer in the situation that created the tensions in the first place. In any event, these tensions are not who you are, but just what you have been experiencing.

When you remove your eyeglasses, you allow your consciousness to *just be* who you really are in the moment of experience. Tensions can then be released from your consciousness and from your eye muscles, allowing your eyeballs to resume their natural shape. Positive changes will occur in your sense of being, as well as your way of seeing.

You'll notice there are times when your vision will be clearer than others. You will also be able to distinguish the differences between the states of consciousness you're in when your vision is clearer and when it's not. After a while, you'll see there's really nothing wrong with your eyes, there's just been something on your mind, and when it's cleared, your vision will be at its naturally clear state, as well.

Clearing your vision accompanies putting your life in order, so that you can again experience calmness.

As your eyeglasses remain off for longer and longer periods of time, your consciousness will be able to relax more and more, and your vision will be clearer and clearer. When you really need your eyeglasses to do whatever you are doing then put them on, and when you are finished, remove them again. If when putting on your eyeglasses you notice a strain, it means that the glasses are already too strong, and getting a weaker prescription would be more appropriate than again allowing your eyes to re-adjust to the glasses. Continue the process until normal vision is recognized, or perfect vision is achieved.

Make sure your optometrist is correcting your vision to normal or slightly less than normal vision. A number of conscientious optometrists like to correct vision to clearer than normal vision. This means that even someone with normal vision would likely be told they need glasses. Their vision would be clearer with the glasses prescribed, but it would be an over-correction, and they would then become dependent upon the unnecessary eyeglasses.

Normal vision is not perfect vision. People with normal vision see clearly most (not all) of the time, and see most (not all) things clearly.

What you are interested in doing is returning to normal vision without your eyeglasses. If you then wish to continue until you experience perfect vision, all well and good, but the important thing is to first release yourself from the dependency you've had on eyeglasses, those prosthetic devices which have become fashion, like canes. You don't need them.

During the period of improvement, there will be 'flashes' of clear eyesight, and another state of consciousness accompanying them with which you can identify. Things will be apparent (clear) during these flashes that were not apparent before. The realizations during the flashes of clarity are reference points that you can remind yourself of when needed in order to consciously recreate the state of consciousness that came spontaneously before. The truth of the revelation for you will be reflected in the clarity of the vision that accompanies the realization. The realization may be "It really is a friendly world," or "I am surrounded by love and beauty," or "It really is all perfect," or "It's safe to be myself." It depends on the reasons you chose to not see, and the accompanying decisions you made about the way the world is ("It's an unfair world," or "Nobody is on my side," etc.). It will be apparent that the old decision was not, in fact, a reflection of truth, but just the way things seemed when seen through a distorting emotional filter. The decision to follow the path of personal truth, rather than defensive distortion or someone else's truth, encourages and accelerates the process of transformation and return to clarity.

These flashes represent the true state of your vision and let you know the experience of clear vision already exists within your consciousness. This means you really can (are able to) see, but have not been identifying with the experience of clear vision. What remains is for you to identify with the clear state of vision, and not consider it extra-ordinary. It is actually your new ordinary state of vision, and the state of consciousness accompanying it is your new ordinary state of consciousness, in which clarity of consciousness accompanies clarity of eyesight. When you do once again experience clarity, you will realize it is not a new state of consciousness after all, but rather your old natural state – before you became unclear. The process is one of remembering, rather than discovering.

These flashes of clear vision show you those times when you have crossed a threshold. Vision improvement often does not proceed as a smooth continuum, but rather in a wave pattern, so there are times of clarity and times of blurriness. It's important to maintain a sense that whatever the state is in the moment of experience, the direction is positive.

You can then remind yourself of the direction – always up!

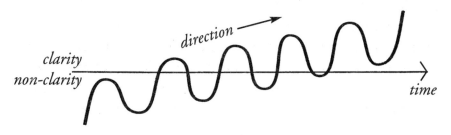

The flashes of clear vision may accompany a realization of what is really true for you, when you had been, in a sense, fooling yourself before. For example, "I never really liked this job, and I knew I should have left before," or "I knew he wasn't right for me," or "She really does love me." Then, the increased clarity could stimulate decisions to make changes in your life.

This is the real you emerging. Start each day with no preconceived notion of who you are, and with a willingness to be real. Your consciousness will automatically reach out and bring to your awareness any information you need to improve your vision, in keeping with your unique beliefs and value systems. It may include mental changes, changes in diet, exercise, insights, and/or new understandings of past experiences. Follow your inner guide.

At the end of the day, you can see who you were in different situations, and how you responded to conditions around you, and examine the effectiveness of these interactions, comparing them with the picture of yourself that you had before, seeing the changes. Some people have found it useful and helpful to maintain a personal journal of the transformation process.

We are told by Beings we consider evolved that we each create our own reality While we may believe them and sense what they say is correct, our thought patterns and ways of speaking often seem to deny this truth. For example, people talk about others 'making' them angry, rather than having become angry in a situation. Some describe how they were 'made' to do something, rather than saying they had allowed themselves to be manipulated. These people are not describing their experience in a way that reflects the idea they have created their own reality.

Most people with impaired vision describe themselves as "not able to see", a statement that does not reflect the idea that they have created their reality. To do so, they would have to say, rather, that they have been keeping themselves from seeing, or avoiding seeing, or avoiding looking at something, and in a deep sense, this is true. It must be evident that to avoid something, or keep from seeing it, one must be aware of it in the first place. Otherwise, how could it be avoided? You might accidentally see it.

Underneath it all, you can see, and you know what it is that you have been avoiding seeing. It has been you, who you really are, and what is real and true for you. If you choose to see that which you have been avoiding looking at, you will be able to, and the truth shall set you free.

Do you see what I mean?

Affirmations

I accept new ways of thinking and seeing which are clearer for me.

I accept what I see, and I see more clearly.

I see clarity coming.

Chapter 3

The Process of Change

For some people, clear vision returns very quickly once they look inside to see who they are and make a decision about what they need to do in order to be happy. For instance, one remarkable case involved a woman who was always putting other people's feelings before her own and as a consequence had been farsighted for years. She saw how a major source of unhappiness in her life had been her marriage and decided to leave her husband. She committed herself to it, and acted on it. One week later, her vision was clear.

For others, an idea rather than an external action can bring clarity – almost like waking from a dream. A nearsighted woman had felt trapped by life and circumstances, but suddenly realized the only person holding her back was herself – her thoughts. She realized that she didn't have to *get* free, she *was* free – she just needed to *be* free. She said, "Oh. Of course," and she saw clearly.

For most people, the process of change is more gradual and connected with changes to be made in their lives. One farsighted woman achieved clarity in two hours, but it only lasted for one hour. During that time she saw the changes she knew she had to make, but was not ready to make. In order to be comfortable she needed to make the changes gradually and harmoniously. She returned to the farsightedness she had experienced for 23 of her 26 years, but with the memory of what she had experienced for that one hour. She did no further work on her vision, but over the next four years changed her relationship, her home, and her job. With each change, her eyesight improved. As each source of conflict or tension was released, her vision improved, until again she experienced clarity – permanently this time!

The process of increasing clarity often (though not always) has three stages of visual change. These stages can take place over hours, weeks, months, or even years, depending on the individual's sensitivities. Most people take weeks or months. Stages one and three are commonly reported by many people on their path to clarity – stage two is less common.

Stage One – Colors

The first stage is commonly noticed as a change in the perception of colors; they seem brighter, as though a gray film has been removed from in front of the eyes. At this stage, the details are not yet clearer, but the colors are. This indicates that at least one of the perceptual filters has been released; a misperception has been released, or some idea which had kept the individual from fully experiencing life has been let go of. At this point, things have already begun to make sense in a different way.

In my experience, this happened just before an operation, when I had been told I might not survive. I went through the emotional stages familiar to anyone who has worked with the dying process. At first it didn't seem real, like it wasn't happening to me. My consciousness looked for a way out, but didn't find one. Finally, I had to consider the possibility that this was actually happening to me. I had to accept the unacceptable.

When I did finally accept what was happening as reality, my body shook. There was a release of energy and the gray film lifted – even though I had not realized it had been there. Not only were colors brighter, all of my senses were also experienced more intensely. I saw how the fear of death had, ironically, kept me from experiencing being alive. Having accepted death, I could fully live.

The process for me was much stronger than most people who are improving their eyesight experience. There is usually none of the intense shaking I experienced. Instead, there is a realization that the colors are brighter, without even knowing exactly when the change happened. However, for those rare times when there is such an intense release, it's helpful to know it is a positive process leading to a rebirth, and a much more fulfilling way of Being. They can then accept the process with more trust. Remembering the word, 'Acceptance,' and what it means to them, is very helpful.

When the brighter colors are experienced, this should be seen as a signal that the process of vision improvement has begun, even though the details one sees may not yet be clearer.

Stage Two – Selective Vision

After the increased clarity of colors, the next stage may be selective vision. The details of the selective vision are different for different individuals, yet the generic process is the same.

Note: It's important to mention here that some people experience this stage, and others may not. In fact, this stage is relatively uncommon, but when it does happen, the individual should be able to understand what is happening, within the context of improving their vision. If it is not experienced, it does not mean the process is not working, but rather it is different for that individual.

Some may notice how if they look at people and objects from the same distance, they see the objects more clearly than the people. This is a selective process in their consciousness, not a problem with their eyes. They realize they have not been seeing something clearly about people. It's not something bad that they have been avoiding seeing, but something good.

For example, one nearsighted woman I worked with had an embarrassing experience in school when she was young and very sensitive. She imagined everyone watching was judging her and her way of being, and this had left her with a fear of people, worrying what others may think of her if they got to know her. What she had been keeping herself from seeing was that people were really on her side, they were not judging who she really was, but rather enjoying and admiring her way of Being.

Selective vision can be used as an inner guide. It's a bit like watching a television where most of the picture is blurred, but some details are clear. You can direct your attention to the clearer parts. Entering a room full of people, you may notice that while most of the people appear blurred, there may be one person, or group, which appears clearer. This shows you where you are 'connected' in the moment. Go over to the person, or group, and see what the nature of your connection is. The point of clarity may change after a while, and then you can migrate to the next place your choice of clarity guides you.

Your consciousness, your Higher Self, is highlighting your path to harmony and clarity. After all, who is it that is making some parts of the picture clearer than other parts? Your Spirit is attracting your attention to what is clear for you. You are being presented with an opportunity to interact with another level of consciousness. Suddenly this becomes not just a process of improving eyesight, but rather developing a relationship with this deeper part of your-self.

An artist in Paris, who had been nearsighted, had spent most of her life seeking acceptance and not perceiving when she was being accepted. As her vision started to improve, she noticed it was clearer whenever she was in one part of the city, rather than another. This was a place where she felt she belonged – where she fit in and did not need to seek acceptance. She also changed her dress style, no longer dressing for other people so that they would take her seriously, but dressing for her own comfort and sense of aesthetics. Her vision improved as she accepted herself for who she is. Her art also changed. Previously, she had mainly painted faces with prominent eyes. Now, more features were developing, and finally she began to paint bodies as well.

The process of selective vision shows how your blurred eyesight is not a reflection of something wrong with your eyes, but rather something on your mind. When the issue is cleared, clarity will return to your sight as well as to your consciousness.

Stage Three – Recognition of Clarity

The third stage is the recognition of clarity, and you know then that you can stabilize your way of Being. The changes are complete and your vision is affirming you are being true to yourself. Of course, you knew that, but the visual feedback reinforces your certainty.

As your vision improves, you may begin to see more clearly around the periphery of what you are looking at; so the point you focus on is not yet clear, but the area around it is. This is a phenomenon known as Eccentric Fixation. As your vision continues to clear, you will notice the clarity migrates closer and closer to the point you are looking at – until it becomes the clearest point in your field of vision. This is called Central Fixation, and is a sign of normal vision. As this external visual process goes on, you will notice a corresponding process in your consciousness; your thinking will be clearer and more focused, too.

By this stage you will have explored your consciousness, released distorting filters that had interfered with your perceptions, and gotten your life to work so much better. You will also know you have achieved a degree of mastery over your own consciousness. As a result, you will have a new dimension of living to explore. If you ever experience non-clarity of vision again in the future, know that it's because something in your mind needs to be resolved, and when that's done, you will again return to your natural state of clarity.

As you experience the changes in your life that accompany the changes in your vision, things will make sense in a different way from before. Some of the ideas and attitudes you had held on to – maybe even defended – will no longer make sense. They were the result of defensive distortion, rather than clarity. Release the old ideas and attitudes in favor of those resulting in greater harmony and improved clarity. Know all these changes are happening for the better. The old ideas and attitudes reflected who you thought you were – not who you are now.

Your vibration will change as you move into a new paradigm. You might release not only ideas and attitudes, but also people and experiences. This is making room for others who are more in accord with your new vibration. You will be looking at your life through new eyes.

Others will notice this difference in you, too. Some may not understand and will be concerned, because they are holding on to the image of who you were, rather than seeing who you really are. If this happens, you can explain that you are going through a process of personal transformation, and that the changes they have noticed are working for you. Tell people you are experiencing more clarity about who you are and that you are getting your life to work better for you.

Anyone willing to encourage the changes can be helpful to you in the process. They can be someone to talk to about what is happening and what is real for you. Anyone who is discouraging and not wanting you to make the changes – preferring to hold on to the picture of you in the past – may attempt to invalidate the process you are experiencing. Know that you don't need to convince them. Just do what feels right for you. After the process is complete, they may see things another way.

Despite the many people who have already improved their vision, and the many organizations dedicated to the process of vision improvement, there are still some who prefer to believe the process of vision improvement does not work. Such people may even want to convince you of this , "for your own good," as their expression of love. This would place you in the delicate position of feeling that you might need to defend the fragile new reality that you have just begun to nourish. Rather than doing this, just explain to these people that you are putting your life in order, for inner clarity. Afterward, you will have the results to show these people, if they are interested.

Trust your path towards clarity, and trust who you really are.

Affirmations

Clarity is freedom, and being real.

As I clear my life, my vision clears.

I am free.

Section II

Using Your Mind
As a Tool

<u>Chapter 4</u>

Create a New Reality

If you see yourself as a success, you are. If you see yourself as a failure, then you are successful at that, too. You are always successful at creating your reality from your perceptions.

Whatever you believe to be true, is true – for you. Your perceptions create your reality. Whatever you believe about people you reinforce and affirm continually, until that's all you see around you. To you it appears to be universal, but in fact it is only so in your field of perceptions, the bubble you are in the middle of. Elsewhere, other things are true, but you do not experience them – other people do.

You may believe, for example, the world is not a safe place, or that you cannot really trust love, or that everyone around you is playing games with love. When something happens that causes you to respond with hurt, you remind yourself of your basic belief. "See – I knew it!" You seem to be a magnet attracting that quality of experience.

Elsewhere though, other people are attracting other qualities of experience. So, what is different about them? They affirm a different reality, and so experience it. Your perceptions predispose you to certain ways of responding to your environment, and you are then assured of a particular way your environment will respond to you.

Right now, you perceive yourself as not being able to see clearly without eyeglasses. Regardless of how you reached this state, it is what you believe to be true for you. And so it is.

When you change your perceptions – so that deep inside you know you can see clearly without eyeglasses – your perceptions will create that reality, and it will be so. Right now, this may seem like a big jump to make. Perhaps you find it difficult to believe you really are capable of seeing clearly now. What you can do, however, is allow yourself to believe that you are getting better and better, and seeing clearer and clearer, until you see that it's true for you.

We can say that you are interested in leaving one reality and entering another, where things are different, and behave differently.

You are involved in the improvement of your vision, and moving from a reality in which you do not experience clear vision, to a reality in which your vision is clear. You know that when you are in the new reality, things will make sense in a different way. You will also experience a different way of Being.

Since your perceptions create your reality, in order to move from one reality to any other there must also be a change in your perceptions.

The process of movement from one reality to another involves three steps:

1. Decide what will be true in the new reality.

2. Encourage the perception that it's happening now.

3. Know you are in the new reality NOW. Decide that now, it's true!

It doesn't matter whether you are moving from unclear vision to clear vision, from illness to health, from poverty consciousness to prosperity consciousness, or from low self-esteem to high self-esteem; the same process applies.

This book can provide the first step, and give you the tools for the second and third steps. It's you, though, who must use the tools in order for them to work. Your consciousness must reach out with a positive sense of expectancy, expecting the process to work for you.

Step 1

What *will* be true in the new reality? You will see more clearly that which you did not see clearly before.

Step 2

Use the tools in this book to help the shift in your perceptions, and encourage the perception that the shift is happening right now. Continue to use the tools until you have reached the third step and no longer need them. Any of the tools used alone may be all that you need. Any combination of tools strengthens the process.

Assure yourself the process of improving your clarity is not something that's *going* to happen, but rather something that is happening *now* – even if you may not yet have noticed the improvement. It is happening *now*. The point of power is always *now*. All changes that happen in your life happen in this moment called *now*.

When you experience even a brief moment of improved clarity, rather than considering it an extra-ordinary state, which may disappear in a moment, use it as evidence that the process is really working now. When you have a positive sense of expectancy, you watch for evidence of success. If improved clarity is considered extra-ordinary, it is, in a way, mentally rejected, and the tendency is to return to the 'ordinary' state of consciousness.

Identify with the clarity and the mental and emotional states associated with it. This is your new ordinary state of consciousness. After a while, not experiencing clarity will be extra-ordinary and you will be able to return with more and more ease to the new ordinary state of consciousness in which you see clearly.

The words you use to describe your experience create your reality. Until now, when you have experienced non-clarity of vision, you have described the experience to yourself as something being wrong with your eyes. After a while, you will see that when you are in one particular mental state, or state of mind, you see more clearly than when you are in another, different state of mind, and you will build a different association. Then, if you do not experience clarity of vision in a particular moment, you will know that it's because there's something on your mind, and when it's cleared, your vision will clear again, and you'll return to your natural state of clarity.

And it will be true for you.

Continue to encourage your improvement process until clarity is stabilized. Consciously direct your attention to notice things you can see more clearly than before, and own the improvement. Insist on noticing increased clarity, however slight, thus reinforcing your perception that the process is working now

Step 3

When your vision is clear and you identify with the state of consciousness you experience as being who you really are, you will know the work is complete. When clarity is identified as your natural state of being, and is what you are experiencing, consider that you may never again experience non-clarity, but now may function normally from a clear space.

You will be aware of the dynamics necessary to maintain balance and clarity. Keep your perceptions in the present, oriented toward the future, and see your past way of Being as the person you have been – the person you were before the return to clarity – and different from who you are now.

You will be able to see your past self with compassion, and understand how you had acted as the result of the perceptions experienced by you at that time. There will be no need to apologize for or defend the actions of a Being that no longer exists, but rather to function with clarity in the present, enjoying your new life, experiencing fulfillment as your natural birthright.

Affirmations

My vision continues to clear
as I adjust to my new state of consciousness.

My vision is improving now.

I notice that I see more clearly every day.

Chapter 5

Positive Thinking

It's imperative that you maintain a positive attitude during the process of change. Positive thoughts are success-oriented. Look for and find a way to change any non-success-oriented thought to one that supports the success you are enjoying. Eliminate the word *can't* from your vocabulary. When you use the word, at some level you are saying there is something you're not able to do. It denies the truth that we are each unlimited Beings, and able to do anything we decide we really want to.

If you can imagine it, you can do it!

If you do find yourself using the word 'can't', then change what you are saying so that you are still expressing what is true for you, yet in a different way. Your thinking will become more precise, and more positive.

Examples

"I can't stand that"   becomes   "I feel resistance to that"

"I can't do it"   becomes   "I haven't yet learned how"

"I can't see that"   becomes   "I don't see that,"
                        or   "I don't yet see that clearly"

"I can't handle that" becomes   "That's been difficult for me
                                        until now"

"I can't remember" becomes   "I don't recall right now, but it
                                 will come in a moment"

"I can't understand" becomes   "I don't understand "

Do the same for non-success-oriented words and phrases:

" It doesn't work"   becomes   "It hasn't yet worked,"

" It isn't working"   becomes   "I haven't yet seen results"

"I don't know how" becomes   "I haven't yet learned how"

"It's terrible"   becomes   "It has got to get better"
              (and notice something positive about "It")

"It's a failure"   becomes   "Success has been temporarily
                                 delayed, and anyway, I learned
                                 something"

Build a pattern of success. Start small – *if you must* – and be successful at it. Reward your successes with congratulations. Reward
only your successes.

Pleasure is positive, too. Pleasure yourself. Give yourself pleasure. Walk on the sunny side of the street. Enjoy the scent of a flower.
Enjoy its beauty. Enjoy what you do see. Enjoy the colors and the
forms, even if you do not yet see the details. As you build more and
more positive habits, you will see more and more benefits and
advantages, and the process will accelerate.

If your picture of yourself is not totally positive, then you are not really seeing yourself, you are only seeing who you think you are, You are only aware of whom you have seen yourself as, in the past. In the reprogramming of your consciousness, leave behind any of the traits or habits that limited you, or that you do not wish to carry into the future. You can acknowledge these traits as having belonged to you, and decide that you no longer need to have them. You no longer need to do those things. You can see a new way of being which works better for you.

Be aware of whether your pictures of the future are positive or not, and always remember to leave the door open for positive change.

For example, saying something like, "Each time I see that person I get a headache," is really saying that each time you saw that person in the past you got a headache, and the next time you expect it to be the same. You are not leaving the door open for positive change. If a headache is not being experienced when meeting that person, it will be expected, and searched for, and then it will certainly come. It would make more sense to say something like, "Every time I've *seen* that person *in the past* I've *gotten* a headache, but next time might be different. Perhaps that person has changed, has realized the error of their ways. It may even be a very positive experience. I'm willing to be pleasantly surprised." This way a positive experience will be anticipated. Seeing the other person in a positive light will also make it easier for *them* to respond differently. Your perceptions create your reality.

Do the same with your own traits. Instead of deciding you won't be able to read that small newspaper print, say that you've not been able to before, but now, let's see. Perhaps now you WILL be able to read that newspaper, or thread that needle, or see that television screen, or write that letter without your eyeglasses or contact lenses.

In fact, you can probably continue to read this book without your eyeglasses or contact lenses, and notice that it gets easier and easier as you go along. Right?

Some say the mind is like a drunken monkey, playful and mischievous when it has nothing to do. When it has something to do, an assignment, it applies itself diligently. So, keep it busy with the idea that your vision is improving and let it find ways of reminding you of this. It will find many. Say to yourself, "I'm seeing clearer and clearer and noticing things I can now see that I didn't see before." Your mind has an assignment and it *has* to prove you're right. You will, in fact, then notice the truth of such statements.

Those times you have been spending talking to yourself in a way that was not particularly useful, and moving from a positive idea (success-oriented) to a negative idea (failure-oriented) and back again – thinking of nothing in particular that was really important or creative – could be spent in another way. You could be reminding yourself of all the ways you are getting better and better, noticing things you can see which you did not see as clearly before, and keeping a positive attitude toward the improvement process. Judgmental thoughts can be replaced with creative thoughts.

Tell yourself how you appreciate your sense of eyesight, and your eyes. They are not 'bad eyes', but wonderful eyes, which had become weak for a while, and are now getting stronger.

Love your eyes.

Love heals.

Notice from how far away you can see the individual bricks on distant buildings, or the leaves on trees, and how that keeps improving. Rather than keeping your thoughts on how weak your vision had been, keep your mental focus forward, on the state of improvement, and how you notice it more and more.

Enjoy your sense of vision. When it is blurred, enjoy the colors, and when it is clear, appreciate the details. If you had been completely blind for a while and were then able to see what you see now, how would you feel about what you see? You would love it, and appreciate it.

Notice the things you think about other people, and ask yourself if they are positive or judgmental thoughts. It is *always* possible to find something positive to notice – so do it. As this becomes more and more a new habit, you'll experience a more relaxed state of being and will find it easier and easier to experience more love in your life.

You can think of someone who loves you, and wants to see you happy and healthy. Notice the good feeling that comes when you think of this person. As you feel this good feeling, this love, remind yourself that love heals. Know that as long as you experience this feeling, healing energy is restoring you to balance on all levels. During your day, you'll be able to think of more and more people in this way, and know the love you feel with these people is having a positive healing effect on your vision. And besides – just feeling all of that love during your day will feel terrific.

Allow the positive changes in your personality to unfold and recognize them. Encourage them. The character traits with which you had previously identified belonged to the old you – and the new you who is emerging is who you really are. Keep the past in the past. Identify only with the positive qualities you notice more and more and the quality of your life, which feels happier and happier as you emerge more and more.

It will be easier if you discuss your vision project only with those who encourage it and would like to see you succeed. Others who do not fully understand the process may try to discourage you, with what they consider good intentions. Wait until you have achieved a noticeable, measurable degree of improvement before discussing it with these people. They will not be able to argue with success.

Constantly hold the idea in your mind that your vision is in a constant state of improvement, and it's happening now. Read at least one chapter in this book each day during the improvement process, and notice how the words make more sense and the ideas become clearer and clearer.

You are on an exciting, magnificent inner voyage through the realms of your consciousness. You are discovering the multi-dimensional nature of your vision, and the relationship between your mind and your body. You are exploring the very nature of your Being, who you really are, the power of your mind and imagination, and what they can do.

What you are discovering is leading you to the knowledge that there is nothing you cannot do, only some things you have not yet learned to do.

Now, you are learning to improve your eyesight and vision, and noticing the improvement more and more. You are discovering more and more that you really can see, and that clarity is your natural state of Being.

Affirmations

Every day, in every way, I'm getting better and better.

Instead of problems, I see solutions. I see the way things can work.

Clearing my vision is easier than I thought!

Chapter 6

Affirmations

What are affirmations?

Affirmations are positive statements that encourage the change, or describe the view from the new reality. You may use the affirmations passively, listening to them often, reading them repeatedly, or thinking about them from time to time. When you use affirmations in this way they will have a subtle yet definite effect. Over a period of time, your consciousness will tend to reach for the way the words make sense Eventually you will see the truth of these words, and the statement – the affirmation – will be a basic belief in your new consciousness.

To accelerate the process, you may also take a more active role in using the affirmations, mentally agreeing with them, and looking for evidence of their truth.

One affirmation, for example, could be, "It's easier and easier to see clearly". To use this actively, when you hear the words, read them, or say them to yourself, direct your attention to your visual field and notice the quality of your vision with a positive sense of expectancy. Notice that it *is* easier for you. Remind yourself that even if it is difficult, as you repeat the affirmation over a period of time it will never again be as difficult, and look forward to the next time, when it will be easier. Soon, you'll notice that it is, indeed, easier and easier to see clearly.

Replace any non-constructive thought with an affirmation. Any time you are thinking idly, remind yourself of the affirmation and watch for evidence of its truth. When you are involved with judgmental thoughts which do not feel good for you, switch channels and think of an affirmation that reminds you of the improvement process, and which feels better.

When the improvement of your vision is the most important thing that is happening for you, your thoughts will tend to return to that process.

When affirmations that describe the view from the new reality are used actively and mentally agreed with totally, the jump to the new reality can be immediate. From that moment, that will be what is true. You may then identify the new reality as your new ordinary state of Being, and discover the other aspects of the new Being that have improved at the same time.

Following is a list of affirmations, with expanded explanations. Choose one affirmation each day and use it often during the day. You will see its effect. The next day, use another. Continue this until you see clearly and no longer need to affirm the improvement process. You will not only know that you can see clearly, you *will* be seeing clearly.

Affirmations that encourage the process of change

1. My vision is improving now.

This means that the improvement of your vision is not something you expect to happen in the future, but something that is happening *now* in your consciousness – something related to the process of improvement. You may or may not have noticed it yet, but it *is* happening now. If you haven't yet noticed it, it's just a question of time before the improvement crosses the threshold of notice-ability.

2. I choose clarity.

The non-clarity of your vision has been the reflection of non-clarity on other levels. You recognize this and affirm your decision to replace non-clarity with clarity on all levels. You are willing to make it a conscious choice in every situation. In any situation that involves choice between clarity and non-clarity, you choose clarity, and what is true for you. You see the benefit of doing this, and others really appreciate it, too. You choose to see what you had avoided looking at before. In the moment of choice – the moment of truth – you choose clarity, and what is real.

3. I know what clarity is, and I experience it more and more each day.

The recognition of non-clarity implies the knowledge of clarity. How could there be the recognition of something being unclear, if you didn't know clarity? You are affirming that this knowledge and recognition of clarity is brought more and more to conscious awareness, and that you identify with it more and more each day, and more and more today.

4. I remember clarity, and I am returning to clarity.

Before your vision became unclear, it was clear. The memory of clarity is in your consciousness. It's not a process of discovering clarity, but rather remembering it and allowing it to return, and recognizing this process as it happens.

5. I notice that I see more clearly every day.

With this affirmation, you are saying that not only do you know your vision is clearer, but you are also reminding yourself of this by noticing what is clearer today than yesterday. You are consciously directing your attention to the improvement process.

6. I know I can see clearly now.

You affirm that you know the ability to see clearly exists within you. You are affirming that you do have the ability to see clearly. Even those times when you do not experience absolute clarity, you know you can – you have the ability – to see clearly. When you experience clear vision, the same words have another meaning. At that time, you know that the experience of clarity is yours. You not only have the ability to see clearly, and know that it exists within you at this time, this is also what you say (*I can see clearly now*) when you are *experiencing* the clarity of vision. This double meaning accelerates the experience of clarity, with anticipation of the evidence of the truth of the statement right now.

7. I know my experiences lead me to clear vision.

You know that at some time in the future you will be experiencing clear vision consistently. You also know that everything you experience between now and then will give you information leading you to that clarity. Even the experience of non-clarity reminds you what clarity is. You are also seeing the relationship between what you experience in your life and what you experience in your vision, and this is also leading you to clear vision, and total clarity.

8. I accept new ways of thinking and seeing which are clearer for me

You recognize that your ways of thinking and seeing have not been clear for you, and affirm your willingness to release these in favor of clarity and to identify with new ways of thinking and seeing. Defensive distortion no longer makes sense – acceptance of clarity does.

9. Acceptance and love lead to clarity.

Emotional acceptance of who you are and what is true for you is an aspect of clarity. It is also a necessary first step in the process of change. Seeing yourself as you are and seeing others as they are allows acceptance, which is love. Releasing the tension of judgments, expectations, and misperceptions allows clarity to return.

10. I accept what I see, and I see more clearly

Anxiety about the quality of your vision increases tension and creates and maintains non-clarity of vision, and so does non-acceptance of the content of your visual field. Emotional acceptance of what you do see releases tension, enhances relaxation, and has a positive effect on your vision. In addition, you are willing to see what is true, and the emotional acceptance of what is true, rather than the denial or resistance to it, also releases tension and allows clarity.

11. It's easier and easier to see clearly.

As you learn more about yourself, it becomes easier and easier to apply this knowledge. Practice with the techniques and ideas also makes them more familiar, and the process of change also becomes more familiar. You affirm that you notice the increasing ease. You will see that returning to clarity is easier than you thought it would be.

12. I'm letting myself be real, and watching my vision clear.

You have been keeping yourself from being real – not allowing it, not giving yourself permission. Now you allow it – in fact insist on it – and you notice your vision clearing as a result. You can just focus on being real and see the effect this has on your vision.

13. It's more and more comfortable to be myself, and to see clearly.

You have not been comfortable with really being yourself; perhaps not trusting it would be all right. As you allow yourself to function more and more from your center – and see that it is indeed all right – you feel more comfortable with that. You are more comfortable also with the clarity of vision which is still new for you.

14. My mind is reaching out and bringing to my awareness any information I need to experience clear vision.

You are giving your mind an assignment, and are willing to see the evidence of its effect. You are affirming trust in the process and you know therefore that whatever information your mind presents to you is related to the improvement of your vision.

15. I can see clearly today.

You have the ability *now* to see clearly, and you realize today might be the day when total clarity of vision is experienced and recognized, and identified with as your natural state. The idea that things must take time is a self-limiting concept, and like all other self-limiting concepts is invalid. There is no reason why it must take longer. Realization can come today. Awakening can come today. You can have clear vision today.

16. Every day, in every way, I'm getting better and better.

This affirms the continuing improvement of your health and your clarity, the return to your natural state of balance and wholeness, and your commitment to seeing the positive aspects of your life. You are realizing more about yourself, resolving issues, working in a positive direction, and seeing positive results. Among other things, your eyesight and vision is also getting better and better.

Affirmations that describe the view from the new reality

17. I see more clearly when I am relaxed and centered.

You notice the relationship between your state of mind and clear vision. You see that one aspect of clear vision – one symptom of clarity – is being relaxed and centered; not just during periods of conscious relaxation, but in a generally relaxed way of Being, with which you are able to identify.

18. I see clearly when I am here now.

You see how the clarity you experience more and more is related to focusing your attention in the present moment of experience, rather than in your thoughts, or in perceptions or preoccupations with the past or future. When you see clearly, you also experience being totally present.

19. Clarity exists here and now.

You see that perceptions of past and future can stand in the way of the clarity of what is happening in the present. You also see you do not have to wait for clarity – it's always available to you now, and you remind yourself of this.

20. Clarity is my natural state.

Clarity is not extra-ordinary; it is your new ordinary state. Non-clarity is not who you are. When you experience clarity, you are experiencing the real you. When you were not clear, you were not being yourself. You now identify with clarity and your return to clarity naturally accompanies your return to balance on all levels, and being who you really are.

21. Clarity is what is true for me.

When you consider an idea and then experience clear vision as a result – even briefly – then you know your clarity of vision shows you your personal truth: what is real for you, and who you really are. You also affirm here that acknowledgment of what is true for you is being clear, and that functioning from clarity is functioning from your natural state, and being who you really are.

22. I enjoy seeing clearly.

When you experience clear vision, you affirm your relationship with it as one of joy. You affirm the pleasure you experience when you see clearly, and you spend more and more time doing what you enjoy. It's an accomplishment of which you are proud, the return of a natural talent that pleases you.

23. I see that everything is working perfectly.

You affirm your vision of perfection. Seeing perfection in your life allows you to see perfection in your field of vision. You are seeing perfection figuratively and literally as this perception releases tensions from your consciousness. You are affirming trust in a positive reality. As you remind yourself of it more and more, you see it more and more.

24. I love when I see clearly.

You affirm not only the joy of seeing clearly, but also the recognition that when seeing clearly, you happen to be in a loving state of

Being. You affirm the connection between the love you feel and the clarity you experience.

25. Clarity is freedom, and being real.

You affirm that being real is being clear, and that not having been real kept you from being free. Being real, and therefore free, you experience clarity. You also affirm the relationship between freedom for others, as well as yourself, and clarity.

26. I see more clearly now.

You see the quality of your vision at this time and notice those aspects of clarity that are related to the degree you focus your perceptions in the here and now. You also affirm that your vision has improved, and you own the improvement. You are also affirming a greater clarity of thought and better understanding than you had previously experienced.

27. I see more clearly than I did before.

You notice the improved clarity of your vision by consciously reminding yourself of the things you can see more clearly now than before. You own the improvement, and you can see particular instances and examples of the improved clarity.

28. Today I choose to see the love.

With this affirmation, you choose to see the love that has always been around you, to which you may not have been paying attention before. When you do this, you also release old perceptions, and see for yourself the effect on your consciousness and vision. You are consciously directing your attention to the love – and the way it's expressed – in all situations you are in and that you see around you during your day.

29. When I do what I really want to do, something wonderful always happens.

You not only affirm the positive effects of being real, you also remind yourself that it's not extraordinary – it's simply the way it is. You trust it more and more, and encourage the process in yourself. You see that you can trust yourself, and that everyone enjoys it and benefits when you do that. Remind yourself of this with each success.

30. I trust being real, and I see clearly.

You affirm here not only the trust in yourself and the positive effects of being real, but also the positive effects on your clarity of vision when you are being true to yourself. You are willing to see what's true for you, and you notice the clarity when you do that. When you see clearly, you notice that you are trusting being real.

Other affirmations

(Write your own thoughts and understandings of what these affirmations mean to you.)

I see clarity coming.

_____

_____

_____

_____

_____

_____

I can notice clear vision today.

_____

_____

_____

_____

_____

As I clear my life, my vision clears.

_____

My vision is clearing now.

_____

I am free!

_____

My vision continues to clear as I adjust to my new state of consciousness.

_____

_____

_____

I see the way things can work.

_____

_____

_____

_____

_____

_____

Clearing my vision is easier than I thought.

_____

_____

_____

_____

_____

_____

I know I can see clearly without eyeglasses.

_____

_____

_____

_____

_____

_____

Affirmation Intensifiers

The following are Affirmation Intensifiers, a special class of affirmation that intensifies the effects of all other affirmations that precede them:

I agree with that statement

or

I agree with those statements

In addition to using one affirmation each day, thinking of it from time to time during the day, and reminding yourself of how it is true, read the entire list once at the beginning of each day, and once at the end of each day, before going to sleep. A condensed list of these affirmations, without the expanded explanations, can be found at the back of this book for quick and easy reference.

At the beginning of each day, when you wake up, let your first thought be an affirmation – any affirmation. You can affirm that today you will notice clearer vision, or that it's possible to see clearly today. By doing this, you will have a positive pre-disposition for the day.

Another Affirmation Intensifier, used before or after each affirmation is:

Affirmations always work

Affirmations

It's easier and easier to see clearly.

I agree with that statement.

Affirmations always work.

Chapter 7

Visualization

What is visualization?

It's the process of imagining or making up pictures in your mind. We do it all the time. Using the idea that when you visualize something, you improve the probability of it happening, we can use this mechanism consciously for healing – or in fact, for creating any future we wish.

With visualization – as with affirmations – there are two primary applications: one is about the end result, and the other is about the means to achieve it.

Seeing the end result

In the process of improving your vision, visualize (or imagine) what it will be like when your vision is clear. Pick a scene that will be true in the future, when your vision is clear. If you are serious about improving your vision, then you must know that at some time in the future your vision will be clear – so what will that be like?

Picture a scene in which you are using your vision in a way you enjoy, maybe watching a beautiful sunset, seeing a movie clearly, noticing the clarity of the details, or easily reading a book or newspaper. Notice that you are seeing clearly without eyeglasses or contact lenses, and enjoying that.

Don't just see the scene as something 'out there,' but rather see the scene through the eyes of the character that you are in the scene. Wear the attitude that it's already an accomplished fact in this scene. It has already happened – in the future. It's like watching a movie where you already know the ending. In fact, the ending is already recorded on the film, even though you haven't yet seen that part.

Example:

Imagine yourself in the future, when your vision is clear, in your eye doctor's office, on a day when the sun is shining, and you're feeling good. You're seeing clearly, and smiling to yourself, because you're imagining the look of surprise on your eye doctor's face when he discovers that you see clearly.

Your name is called and you eagerly go in for the examination. You know that you can see, because you are seeing clearly.

During the examination, you see the eye chart more clearly than ever before. Then you notice the look on your eye doctor's face. It's exactly as you imagined it would be. You hear him say, "I don't understand this, but your vision is much clearer than the last time we examined it. Perhaps we made a mistake with your vision prescription, because it's definitely too strong for you now."

You thank your eye doctor, and know that you are living a scene that you have created.

Note: As you imagine more and more this scene in the future, you move more and more to its fulfillment.

Seeing the means.

You may do this on the physical and/or the perceptual level. Ask yourself, what will be the physical means to the improvement of your vision? What will be happening on the physical level, for example with the eye muscles? And what changes in your perceptions will be happening during the improvement process?

Physical means:

You know that tension in certain eye muscles is associated with your type of impaired vision. A diagram of the eye and the particular muscles associated with errors of refraction can be found earlier in this book. Spend some time each day picturing these eye muscles, and/or feeling them, and imagining them relaxing just a little bit more, and picturing the eyeballs changing shape just a little as the tension is released and they return more and more to their natural shape – perfect for normal vision. Imagine that after you are done, the eyeball and eye muscles are just a bit more their natural shape than they were when you started, and the next time you do this visualization begin from this new improved state. Work with what you can allow yourself to believe is possible, always insisting on knowing that the improvement is there, either just noticeable, or just below the level of notice-ability, but there nevertheless. Give yourself the benefit of the doubt. Know that the improvement is there. You will see the evidence of it more and more.

Perceptual means:

What you are dealing with, after all, are only perceptions – subjective aspects of your conscious experience. You can imagine that you do, after all, see clearly the blurry picture you perceive. It's as though between you and what you are looking at there exists a diffusing screen through which you see the image of whatever is on the other side. You do very clearly see the diffused image – so you can identify with seeing clearly, even while you are not yet experiencing clear vision. Spend some time each day polishing the diffusing screen just a little, or peeling off a thin layer of it, so that you clearly see the image just a tiny bit less diffuse – in other words, just a tiny bit more clear. Again, work with what you can allow yourself to believe is possible, and give yourself the benefit of the doubt. Know the improvement is there, either just noticeable, or just below the level of notice-ability, yet there nevertheless. Next time you do this visualization, begin from the new improved state.

Continue until full clarity is experienced.

Affirmations

I see more clearly than I did before.

*My mind is reaching out and bringing to my awareness
any information I need to experience clear vision.*

I know I can see clearly now.

Chapter 8

Metaprogramming

Metaprogramming is the process of reprogramming your mind to create new perceptions and belief systems in order to create a new reality: a new paradigm. It is a particular application of the use of affirmations, using deep relaxation as a vehicle for planting the ideas deeply in your consciousness.

One very effective way to induce particularly deep states of mental relaxation, which will have a beneficial effect on vision, is by using physical relaxation. As the body relaxes, the mind enters deeper and deeper states of relaxation.

As your body relaxes, and you mind relaxes, and your eyes relax, your brain wave frequency will change from your normal range (known as Beta, 14 to 21 cycles per second), to a more relaxed range (Alpha, 7 to 14 cycles per second). In the Alpha frequency, you are in a more creative state of mind in which visualization is easier and the effects more profound, and in this state you can choose to allow a heightened state of suggestibility to those concepts which are to your benefit and serve your purposes. Learning is accelerated and the ability to visualize is enhanced. The effectiveness of this visualization, as well as of the affirmations you use, is also enhanced enormously.

At this level of consciousness, your mind has greater control over your body (witness the remarkable physical feats of yogis, who function normally at Alpha), and your body can more easily respond to a reality your mind creates. Your experience of this state – which is not a trance state – may be just very relaxed, or more relaxed than you were before, or you may experience slight movement of the eyelids or eyeballs (REM – Rapid Eye Movements).

Metaprogramming can be passive or active.

Passive metaprogramming involves allowing yourself to be guided to deep levels of relaxation and hearing the affirmations, possibly without even having the experience of listening to them. In other words, it may feel as though you are asleep, yet part of your consciousness will hear the words nevertheless and they will have their effect. Listening to a guided relaxation cassette while sleeping is a good example of passive metaprogramming. A deeper experience of metaprogramming may be allowed with hypnosis, during which individuals permit themselves to be guided deeper than Alpha, into Theta (4-7 cycles per second) for even stronger impact.

Active metaprogramming involves you guiding yourself to deeper levels of consciousness – with awareness – and then reminding yourself at these levels of the affirmations you are using. While doing this, look for and find ways of agreeing with these statements, seeing how, in fact, the statements are true. You may also allow yourself to be guided, yet maintain awareness so that you may still consciously agree with the statements. This would be a form of *semi*-active metaprogramming.

At the back of this book are some metaprogramming exercises for you to use (see Section IV – 3. Progressive Relaxation). You can record them onto a cassette, with relaxing music or nature sounds in the background for passive or semi-active metaprogramming. When you become very familiar with the exercises you can guide yourself without the help of a tape – that is, if the improvement process is not yet complete by then!

While positive thinking is applied at all levels and states of consciousness, affirmations and visualizations are particularly effective when done in a relaxed state of consciousness, which can be any state of consciousness more relaxed than what you consider 'normal' for you. Therefore, before doing these techniques, take some moments to place yourself in a more relaxed state of consciousness.

Relaxation Places

How you choose to relax is personal to you. I would recommend a seated position – so you are less likely to fall asleep. Sometimes simply sitting still and counting down from 10 to 1, feeling yourself relax more with each number, is enough. It's a bit like taking an elevator to deeper and deeper states of mind, with the descending numbers showing you the level of relaxation achieved. This takes you to a particular level, a 'place' of consciousness that you decide is perfect for these exercises. You may find that taking three slow, deep breaths and feeling yourself relax more with each exhale accomplishes the same thing, and leaves you in the same 'place.' Either way, you will know that now, working in your 'place,' these exercises will be particularly effective.

You may also remember the most relaxing place you have ever been, or that you can imagine, and then imagine yourself there, feeling the relaxed state of mind being there. This, too, can be used as your 'place.' It's helpful if you always go to the same "place," so that you can identify more and more with the state of consciousness and how it feels more and more real for you.

To guide yourself to even deeper levels of consciousness, which are even more relaxed, for the purposes of metaprogramming, you may use physical relaxation to bring about a state of mental relaxation. You may start by closing your eyes, and then relaxing your toes, then your feet, then your ankles, and so forth, until you have physically relaxed each part of your body up to and including your scalp.

By the time you have relaxed your scalp, you will be more relaxed than you were before. Tell yourself at that time that you are in a more relaxed state of mind, perfect for reprogramming your consciousness with optimal effectiveness. Since the words you use to describe your experience create your reality, it will be so.

Then you may use the affirmations and visualizations that feel most appropriate.

Afterwards, remind yourself that when you open your eyes again, you will notice clearer vision than before. Anticipate the improvement, and notice it, even if it is there for only a brief moment, or is barely noticeable. For you, though, the change will probably be distinct and lasting.

Open your eyes, and notice how much clearer you see.

As you continue to spend some time each day in a relaxed state of mind, you will notice a positive cumulative effect over a period of time. You will notice yourself having a more relaxed way of being and interacting, and a greater sense of aliveness. You will experience yourself being more centered, and you will also be releasing the long-term accumulated effects of stress. You may notice that symptoms not directly related to your eyesight are also diminishing and disappearing as you return to balance on all levels.

You are using your mind as a tool to change itself, to propel you through the process of changing your perceptions at many levels. Notice the changes. Anticipate them. Give yourself every opportunity to experience them. Welcome them.

When you understand something, say, "I see." When something makes more sense, say, "It's clearer now." Notice the increased mental clarity, and the more positive outlook you have on your life. You'll see more and more clearly, at every level, and you'll love the changes in yourself, and in what you see in the world around you.

Affirmations

I see more clearly when I'm relaxed and centered.

I'm letting myself be real, and watching my vision clear.

I enjoy seeing clearly.

Chapter 9

Talk to Yourself

The most vital part of the improvement process will be assuring yourself constantly that your vision is improving, until you know it. It involves talking to yourself a lot – after all, sometimes it's the only way to have an intelligent conversation!

In terms of the creation of a new reality, you have already set an intention and decided what will be true in the new reality – your vision will be clearer. That's the first step of the three mentioned in Chapter 4. Now you must continue to encourage the perception that it's happening now (Step 2) until you *know* it is true and the process is complete for you (Step 3).

Knowing is a state of mind, a sense of certainty that does not require external evidence for its existence, but only a decision in one's consciousness.

There are two different senses of 'knowing' that we can relate to. The first is knowing that the process is working, and under way, and that the end result is assured.

The second sense of knowing is knowing when the process is complete and requires no more reinforcement. Evidence in the outer world can be used to trigger this – such as the result of an eye examination.

To trigger and maintain the first sense of knowing, you must continue to encourage the perception that it's happening now, not just in your thoughts (because living in your thoughts alone will keep you from experiencing the now moment), but also in relationship with what is happening around you.

In your thoughts, you will be processing positively, finding reasons to assure yourself more and more in the success of your program. You might be saying to yourself things like:

- **If other people can do it, I can also.**
- **We all have the same basic equipment – a consciousness – that will do whatever we program it to do.**
- **If it's been done once, it can be done again.**
- **What one person can do, any other person can do.**
- **It's not a question of whether I can do it, but rather *how* I can do it.**
- **I have the tools and I am doing it now.**

As you do this more and more, your sense of certainty will continue to increase. It's also important, however, to see what is happening around you now – in the constant now in which you live during your day – and to use things you do in the now to positively program your mind.

Eating, for example, can be used as a positive programming tool. You can assure yourself , "My body has asked me for this food, through my appetite, so this food must be what my body needs as nourishment for the improvement of my vision. It probably contains exactly the vitamins and minerals necessary for the improvement process, or my body would not have asked for it. This food is helping me see more clearly. My body always asks for exactly what it needs. As I listen to it, I accelerate the healing process. Each person's needs are different, and my body needs this food now. As I enjoy this food, it's easy for my body to get what it needs, and use it. Each act of eating makes me healthier, and able to see better."

As you eliminate waste products from your body, you can tell yourself, "Unnecessary waste products and toxins are now being released from my body, and my body is returning to its natural state of balance. My natural elimination system is working perfectly, and each act of elimination is therefore resulting in greater health and improved clarity of vision."

Whatever you do during your day, you can remind yourself, "This is something that's helping me see clearer." When you are just relaxing, you can remind yourself, "This relaxation is what I need right now. As I relax, my thoughts become clearer, and stress and tension are released from my body and my consciousness, and also from the muscles around my eyes, which have held too much tension. Each moment of relaxation therefore is helping me to be healthier, and see better. I will be able to see things in a more relaxed, more positive way. In fact, I am seeing things in a more relaxed, more positive way now."

As you enjoy what you do see, you can have a sense of appreciation for your sense of vision, rather than resentment. You can say, "That's really a lovely painting I'm looking at now," or, "I love the way she looks. What lovely hair." Direct your attention to things you enjoy seeing, rather than what you do not enjoy. You can say, "I love to watch children playing," or, "This architecture fascinates me," or, "What a lovely color that wall is," or, "I look terrific today." Appreciate your sense of vision.

Talk to yourself to bring yourself more into each present moment, each here and now. You can say, "I feel safe here. I feel free to be myself and do what I want," or, "It really feels great to be with these friends," or, "Here I am. What do I really want to do now? What's real for me? What is this moment offering me?" And then be fully present, in the present moment.

In terms of situations that had been difficult for you, you can say, "I will not be ruled by past prejudices or judgments. I'm willing to take a fresh look, and see what's true now. After all, I need a fresh view. I'm open to new perceptions, and new ways of seeing. I'm willing to see what's true for me now, not from what someone tells me, but only from my direct experience now." Remember, when someone tells you something, you don't know whether it is, in fact, true – only that they say it's true. It is your direct experience that tells you what's true for you.

All of your thoughts and all the words you speak should be encouraging the process you are going through. When you have a goal which is, for a time, the most important thing in your life, then all events around you are in some way related to the fulfillment of that goal. What remains is for you to remind yourself of this, to bring awareness to the process. Notice consciously that what is happening around you is a response to something that you have asked for in your consciousness.

It's a bit like lucid dreaming – walking through a dream, with an awareness that you are dreaming. At first, there is an awareness of the dream personality (yourself), the personality of the character in the dream. You seem to be watching a dream story that is the product of another consciousness, but of course it's just another aspect of your own consciousness – the consciousness of the dreamer. You as the dream personality are able to communicate with the dream by saying, for example, "Okay, dream that I'm watching, I know you are a product of my consciousness. I would like to see you change so that *this* happens." The dream responds by changing, according to whatever you allow yourself to believe is possible, until you are watching the dream unfolding the fulfillment of your wish.

At times, the dream seems to be offering you things you had not consciously asked for, but what you can see will make you very happy, asking you, in effect, "Would you like this?" Then, you can respond to the dream by saying, "Yes, thank you." The dream has taken on the dimension of another Being you are in communication with, another level of intelligence. Dialog with this other intelligence results in a feeling of never being alone, of always having a Being with you with whom you can talk, a benevolent Being who is always on your side, and who is always vitally interested in your happiness, well-being, and fulfillment. Since the dream you are watching is the product of your own consciousness, it is another aspect of you, your own higher consciousness, although many people externalize the personification by calling this other consciousness Universal Consciousness, or God, or Holy Spirit. It is a deep part of your own Being, as you recognize more and more as you continue to communicate with It.

As you watch more and more the relationship between your

thoughts and wishes inside, and the dream outside, you will develop more and more a sense of trust in the direction of the dream, and in your actions through it. Fear and guilt become invalid processes that no longer make sense, and the spiritual nature of your Being will become more evident. You are then able to see your real intentions, and know that everything that has happened in your life has been part of a perfect process of unfolding that which you have really wished for. The perfection becomes evident.

Then, you can see the dream personality (yourself) from the other point of view, from the point of view of the dream (or your Spirit), and see your personality with its formerly limited view, with compassion, and a greater understanding of its sensitivities. You can then see other Beings in the same way, each moving in their respective dreams, living the fulfillment of what had been deep decisions in their consciousness. You can see them with more compassion and understanding, interacting with each other in a very complex, yet perfect, mechanism. With the new view, old tensions brought about by non-understanding disappear from your consciousness and your body. Clarity and balance can return on all levels.

You will see.

Affirmations

I see that everything is working perfectly.

I know that my experiences lead me to clear vision.

*My vision continues to clear as I adjust
to my new state of consciousness.*

Section III

Another Way
of Seeing

Chapter 10

Owning Your Power

Owning your power – your power to be who you really are and to live your own truth – is also about owning your freedom to be yourself. In many ways, you have been giving away your power and freedom by your ways of speaking, thinking and being – usually in order to feel loved and approved of. You have been putting yourself under the control of others, through your words, even in your thoughts, and your behavior.

For example, when you say or think something like, "That person makes me angry," you have given the power and freedom to decide when you are angry to that person. This is like saying you are powerless and this other person has the power to decide when you will be angry. You can choose to not do that any more. It would be more appropriate to say something like, "I get angry when that person does that." In that way, you get to see that you are the one who has decided to be angry, and also that you can choose to feel that, or something else.

No one but you can 'make you' feel angry, sad, depressed, happy, sexy, bored, or anything else. Since you are now in the process of deciding for yourself about your life – your choices, actions, feelings, and what you see – why not own your decision-making power on all levels?

Be aware of the words you use, because they do form the basis of your thought patterns. Listen to your words (internal and external), and notice whether they reflect your freedom to decide for yourself what you feel or do.

How have you given your power away?

Have you been saying, "Let me do this," asking for permission, or have you been expressing your desires by saying, "I would like to do this," or even "I am going to do this?" Have you been saying, "That person manipulated me," or "I allowed myself to be manipulated?"

Have you kept yourself from expressing what you really wanted to because of what you thought someone else would think? Then you have given control of your power of speech to that person.

Have you kept yourself from looking at something or someone because of what another person might think? Then you have given your freedom of choice to see what you want, your power of eyesight, to that person.

Have you kept yourself from doing what you want because of what another person might think? Then you have given away your freedom of action.

If you can relate to the above, you have kept yourself from speaking, from acting, from seeing what was real for you. Whatever you have been doing that has not been working for you, you can choose to not do any more. Clear vision is related to allowing yourself to be real, and trusting that – in fact, insisting on that.

You are free, you know

In owning your freedom, you must also be willing to recognize others' freedom. No one gives you your freedom – it's already yours. It's just up to you to be free. In the same way, you do not give others their freedom. You may only acknowledge that they have it.

When you do or say something, others are free to feel about it as they choose. For you, though, you are just being real, and acting with love and freedom as your motivations. If you are misunderstood, then you can choose to clear things through communication. It is not necessary for you to change your way of Being because of the way another feels. If you do choose to change, it must be because you want to do things another way.

In the same way, if another person does something and you choose to not feel good about it, that's also your choice – they, too, are free. If the not-good feeling is the result of a misunderstanding, it can be cleared through communication. Don't assume anything. Ask, and then you will know.

If the not-good feeling is the result of attachments you need to release on your path to clarity and freedom, you can find another way of thinking and feeling that feels better for you, one in which you are not deciding what the other person should do differently, but rather what you need to do differently. If you expect the other person to change because of the way you feel, then you want to control that person. Do you want to be controlled? Are you willing to stop controlling?

No matter what you do, or say, some people will approve, and others will not. You have the freedom to decide which people to be with. If you choose to be with those who judge you, then you may feel like a weed in a garden, constantly feeling as though you need to defend yourself and your way of Being. You can choose instead to be okay with being judged, knowing you're just being you and others are free to feel what they like. They may be judging you by their standards, but you are living by your own standards. Of course you can also choose to be with people who do not judge you, people who appreciate you for who you are. You can then feel freer, and more relaxed about being real, being who you really are. You'll see that you weren't a weed, but rather just a flower in the wrong garden.

Perhaps in the past you've tended to change yourself, to be someone different from who you really are in order to get love, to be loved. If you would like to know that you're loved for who you are, then you have to be who you really are, and let that image – your real self – be loved.

Love cannot be solicited. It must flow freely, and be freely given. Only then can you know it's real. If you create an image in order to be loved and people love the image, you still do not feel loved for who you really are. If the expressions of love are solicited, then you do not really know whether they would be there if you did not ask for them. You would still not be sure of the love. Notice when expressions of love come freely from others, when you're being real. Then, you'll know that they come because the others choose to express their love, and you'll know it's real. When you know the love is there, open to it, and feel it.

Know too that expressions of love are sometimes misunderstood, because we've all been taught different ways of expressing the love we feel. The way some people express their love is sometimes misunderstood as love being taken away. The misunderstandings can be resolved through communication, so expressions of love afterwards can enhance the experience of the person receiving them, something that feels good for them.

Remember to express your love in that way, too. Express your love in the way you would like others to express their love with you; in a way that results in their feeling good, and a way you would be happy to be on the receiving end of.

You have the power and freedom to be who you really are, to be where you really want to be, with whom you would really like to be (if they would like to be with you), doing what you would really like to do. Others, too, have the same power and freedom.

If you find yourself not honestly able to say, "I love where I am, I love who I'm with, and I love what I'm doing," then something has to change. You have the power and freedom to make that change.

If it's a situation in which you do not feel happy, you have three choices:

- Change the situation. Re-arrange it.
- Change the way you see the situation.
- Leave the situation. Find another.

For example, if the situation is your job, you can change it so that you're doing something there that's more meaningful for you. Or, you can look at it in another way that feels better for you so that you feel happy in it (but it must be real for you). If you do not do either of these, then perhaps you need to be doing something different, in a different job, so that you can look forward each day to spending time and energy there.

If it's your home, does it feel like home to you? If not, re-arrange it so that it does. Otherwise, choose to see it as really perfect for you right now. Otherwise, move.

If you believe these changes are too vast or radical for you, that you 'can't' make them, you have given away your power and freedom. It is not true that you cannot make the changes, but rather that you have chosen not to, for whatever reason you consider valid. You still have the power to create your life the way you would really like it to be and to change what has not been working for you, to change that which has not resulted in your being as happy as you would like to be.

Do you find yourself with people you do not really enjoy being with? If so, you have given away your power to be happy to them. You don't have to do that any more.

If you have given away your power, you can take it back. It's still yours. Own it.

Personal power and freedom also applies to your patterns of thinking and behaving. Recognize those thoughts that have not been optimal, those resulting from misperceptions and limited ways of seeing.

Your attachments and addictions stand between you and freedom. When you are free, you are able to decide in each moment what you would like to do. You do not allow yourself to be controlled by past programs.

While we may think of addictions in relation to substances, and attachments within a different context (things, emotions, etc.), they are conceptually the same. When you are addicted to something, and you don't get it, you don't feel good. The degree to which you don't feel good shows the degree of your attachment or addiction. You can choose to not give your power to your attachments, or to the objects of your attachments. Non-attachment is freedom.

Non-attachment is not detachment. Detachment is removal of

all feelings. Non-attachment allows positive feelings of joy for what you have. When there's something you *don't* have, you are able to focus your attention on what you *do* have. For example, if you are attached to having a lobster dinner, and you don't get one, you are not free to enjoy what you do have. When not attached, you can enjoy a salad, or a steak, or a sandwich, and if you have a lobster, really enjoy it, too.

Being attached or addicted to a person also prevents you from enjoying the moment. When you're with that person, you spend time worrying about when you will not be with them and miss the pleasure of the moment. When you are not together, you spend your time missing them rather than being present with the people you are with. That isn't freedom!

You have the power and the freedom to be totally present wherever you are, enjoying whatever is happening. Lobster dinner or sandwich – alone or not.

Others do not have to change their way of Being because of your attachments, and you don't have to change your way of Being because of the addictions of others. You take total responsibility for yourself, everything you think, do, and say – and acknowledge others have the responsibility for everything they choose to think, do, or say.

Avoid the temptation to decide what other people think, or may do in any given situation, because you don't really know –that's their responsibility. You just need to examine your own consciousness, and what happens in it.

Others are free to want what they want, and you are free to say yes or no to that. It's okay for them to want, and it's okay for you to not want. In the same way, you are free to want what you want, and they are free to want or not want the same thing. When you both want the same thing, there is free agreement, and then something can happen. Otherwise, you can agree to disagree, and each of you can find happiness and satisfaction in your own respective ways.

Everybody is entitled to their own opinion and to their own

thoughts and wishes – and you are free.

Review your life movie, the one in which you are not only the star, but also the director. Be the audience, too. What were the effects of your actions and words? Could you have written a better script for yourself? If so, what would you have done differently? Could you have acted with more love, more understanding? Replay parts of the movie in your mind, doing it differently, and see the different ending. If you prefer the new ending, then next time a similar situation presents itself you can act it out the new way. Dedicate yourself to the decision. Then, you have changed yourself for the better, because it was your choice, and you've learned what you needed to.

Accept the past. Realize that things happened the way they did, with the chemistry of the people involved, in order to have the result that needed to happen. Next time, however, you'll be able to achieve the same result more harmoniously.

Go over your movie until you are honestly able to give it and the leading character great reviews. If you saw that movie in a theater, you would have thought it a fabulous movie, with an inspirational star – you! You would have recommended the movie to your friends, and enjoyed seeing it again.

Notice what your reasons are for doing things. What are your motivations? In a given situation, do you make the fear choice or the freedom choice? Are you doing things because that's what you really choose to do, or are you doing things (or not doing things) because of fear? Trust your instincts, decide what's real for you, and do what you really want to do.

Did you keep yourself from being who you really are because you thought you had to, and find out afterwards that you didn't really have to? Then the basis for your decision and your action were fear and illusion. Make a decision that you don't have to do that any more. You can be who you really are, and people will enjoy you even more. When you do what you really want to do, something wonderful always happens.

Is love your motivation, or is it guilt? Do you do things to avoid feeling guilty, because you would feel guilty not doing them? Or do you act clearly, doing what you really want to do, as an expression of love?

If you have been having fear or guilt as your motivations, do you want to continue that way? You don't have to, you know.

You can make a conscious choice – a deep decision – to no longer have fear, guilt, or anger controlling your life, but rather to act as a free conscious Being. Once you do that, from that moment on, if you discover that your decision to be a certain way, or do (or not do) a certain thing is based on fear, guilt, or anger, you dedicate yourself to making a different decision. Then, you are not allowing yourself to be controlled by past patterns of being or doing, but really living your freedom.

You really are free. You just have to own your freedom, and be free. Not only will you feel better and enjoy your life a lot more, but you will also be releasing patterns associated with your old impaired vision. You will truly be returning to clarity.

You're free to think the way you choose, love the way you choose, and act the way you choose.

People who love you enjoy seeing you happy the way you really like to be happy, being the fullest expression of your Being, being real and being all that you can be. People who love you really want to see you being successful.

It's up to you, though.

You have the power and the freedom to be real, to be happy, successful, and fulfilled. See clearly what is real for you – and live it.

While we've been taught that it's a good thing to be ourselves – necessary, in fact – we have also been taught in so many ways that we have to not be ourselves in order to please other people, and that it's a good thing to please other people, to make others happy. It then seems to be a choice between making others happy, on the one hand, and being ourselves, making ourselves happy, on the other hand. If you have been choosing to not be yourself so others could be happy, you have decided that pleasing others is more important than really being yourself. That may have been a beautiful expression of your love, but at a high cost to you, and your ease of being, and your health. Ease of being is associated with health. Not being yourself requires an investment in energy, which is also known as stress, an unhealthy element from anyone's point of view.

What makes more sense is to shift your priorities so that being real is more important. It is a necessary part of any healing process. You can still enjoy expressing your love in any way that works for you, and yet knowing the importance of being real, being yourself – all the time – with clarity and love.

Affirmations

When I do what I really want to do,
something wonderful always happens.

I trust being real, and I see clearly.

Clarity is what is true for me.

Chapter 11

Your Relationship with Yourself

When relationships are harmonious, things feel good. When they are not, the result is stress. Stress creates symptoms. Harmony releases them, and allows a return to balance on all levels.

If your Self were another person, consider how you would describe your relationship with your Self. To live free from stress, your relationship with your Self must be harmonious. Some people fight with themselves. Some are afraid to be alone with themselves, or are ashamed of themselves, hating themselves. Some people criticize themselves, beating themselves up, or hide from themselves. Some punish themselves, being hard on themselves.

Some people are happy with themselves. They appreciate themselves. They talk to themselves in a positive way, and find ways to please themselves. They let themselves play. They like to let themselves have fun. They accept themselves. If they are hurt, they decide to heal themselves.

Making yourself ill is an act of self-aggression, of self-punishment – though it often comes disguised with a feeling of protecting yourself from something. In this case, the protection mechanism no longer serves the organism, and in fact, from the point of view where we each create our reality, the individual is causing him/herself pain and discomfort. When there is some sort of physical symptom, the body is saying to the consciousness within it, "This is what you have been doing to yourself."

We do to ourselves literally what we have been doing to ourselves figuratively.

What would you say about your relationship with yourself? How has it been?

If your vision has not been clear, you have been keeping yourself from seeing something. You have been hiding something from yourself, or denying what was real and true for yourself. You have been keeping yourself from being yourself. You have not been accepting yourself. Your relationship with yourself has not been terrific.

You have now begun to change that by deciding to heal yourself. If you have dedicated yourself to this process, your relationship with yourself will continue to flourish and improve.

You are involved in a process of self-healing, an expression of love to yourself. The better the relationship with yourself, the easier the return to harmony. If your relationship with yourself is not good, you are likely to be hurting, punishing, or causing yourself pain and discomfort in some way. Your actions will be based on self-denial, rather than expressions of love to yourself.

When your relationship with yourself is harmonious, you find ways to please yourself, to feel good, to do things which result in your success and happiness. The result is health and harmony.

If your relationship with yourself has not been harmonious, don't punish yourself about it. Doing so would just continue the non-harmonious nature of your relationship. Instead, recognize the things that have not been reflections of harmony, and change them. Now.

Make a decision, a promise to yourself, to affirm a positive relationship and change any part of your way of Being that has been causing you pain and discomfort. Resolve those issues if and when they become visible, and affirm that from this moment your actions will be reflections of a decision to be in harmony with your Self.

When you are in harmony with your Self, you do things that make you happy, and you stop doing things that make you unhappy. You do things that please you, and stop doing things that pain you. The result is a sense of feeling good about yourself, and who you are, and filling more and more of your day with good feelings and pleasurable experiences. You *can* feel good all the time. It is possible, and achievable. What it takes is just for you to go for it, and see how much you can achieve. It may take some time, but if you are going to be here anyway, it's just a matter of how you will spend that time. This is one investment in time that will result in dividends of pleasure. We can see it as the economics of harmony.

First, ask yourself a question – how much of your day do you spend feeling good, and how much do you spend not feeling good? Something will have to change about the things that feel not-good.

What is the biggest source of unhappiness in your life? How much time do you spend thinking about that thing? Something must change in that area if you want to be happy. You're going to have to do something about it. The sooner you begin, the sooner you will be happy. You can handle the big ones first, and then ask yourself the same question – what is now the biggest source of not-good feelings in your life? Handle that one next.

You can also decide to begin with the little ones first, the easy ones, and build a pattern of success, gaining momentum for The Big One.

Whether you start with the biggest source of unhappiness or the smallest, the result will be a more relaxed, happier way of Being – and better health! You will also be allowing yourself to be real.

Look at the experiences during your day as being within boxes of time and notice the feelings you have afterwards, compared to the feelings before the experience. Are they the same, or better, or not as good?

If you notice that with a particular kind of experience, you consistently feel not as good afterwards as you did before, you know that you must stop entering that kind of experience if you want to be happy. That experience is standing between you and happiness, and it's not worth your health. It's best released from your life. For example, notice how you feel before reading a newspaper, and after. If you realize that you consistently feel worse after reading newspapers, stop reading them. You will be freeing some time that you can invest in some other activity that has greater dividends of good feelings.

Do this with each activity during your day.

In addition to noticing the feelings before and after the activity, also notice the feelings during the activity. There are some activities that result in good feelings afterwards, yet do not feel great during. There must be another way to achieve the same end, and during which you are able to spend more time feeling good. For example, some massages are quite painful and uncomfortable, yet we subject ourselves to the experience if we believe some good comes from the pain. On the other hand, there are other kinds of massage which feel absolutely delightful, and which have the same benefit.

Eliminate the investments in time that result in negative dividends, and re-invest in pleasure.

Make your choices conscious acts of self-love. Before making any decision about what to do, say, "I love myself, therefore..." then make the choice that reflects self-love.

At first, in deciding what to do, your choices may be about 'the lesser of the two evils,' or making the choice that feels less not-good. Afterwards, the choices are more between what feels good and what feels not-good. Finally, the choices are between what feels great and what feels terrific.

You see more and more the economy of the time you spend, and the quality of experience within that time. You can be happy all of the time.

There may still be 'highs' and 'lows,' but as time goes by you will notice more and more how the 'lows' are where the 'highs' used to be. After a while, even on your worst days, you feel better than you used to feel on your best days. The overall direction is up, continually getting better and better. Instead of seeing the lows as the crashes after the highs, you can see the lows as the catapult to the next high. If it really feels low, think of how great the next high will be!

Be good to yourself in all you do. Let yourself see the love around you in all situations. Spend your time in situations that feel good. Let yourself have exactly what really makes you happy. Be honest with yourself.

In terms of what feels good, look not only at circumstances around you in your physical life, but also at thought processes within you. Decide to choose thoughts and perceptions that feel good for you, and also result in good feelings. Remember to always acknowledge what is true, and what is true for you. By doing so, you can see what feels good for you and what does not. You can stop doing those things that don't feel good, leaving more time during your day for pleasure.

As you continue to do this, life will become more and more pleasurable for you, and you'll experience less stress. It will become a new habit. Your life will become more and more consciously motivated towards pleasure, and you'll have a chance to examine your relationship with pleasure. If you have been denying yourself, you will be able to indulge yourself. You will begin to feel more and more good about feeling good, recognizing it as an organic process, one that supports life.

You will be able to recognize that the natural order of the universe is harmony, and pleasure. When you experience something different from that, it's a signal that something is wrong – out of order. The recognition will enable you to re-orient yourself, and get on with your life in a positive way. As you experience more harmony, your consciousness will be clearer and clearer, and so will your vision.

• As you accept yourself more and more, without judgment, you'll also become more and more able to accept others, and more perceptual filters will lift. You will trust yourself more and more, and allow yourself to exist more and more in the present moment of experience – the here and now – where your vision exists, and is most clear.

• As you return to balance in your consciousness, the rest of your organism on the physical level will return to its natural state of balance. You will be able to experience your natural state of clarity on all levels.

It's not just all right to be happy – you're supposed to be happy – if you want to be healthy.

When you create a sense of harmony within yourself, it's as though you exist in a clear bubble, with everything else and everyone else outside the bubble. Within this clear space, you can clearly direct your thoughts to anything or anyone, or you can withdraw again into the bubble, and the clear space you experience within it.

As you direct your thoughts to a subject, notice your feelings, and whether they are totally clear, or whether your instincts are showing you a feeling that doesn't feel totally clear. Release the subject from your thoughts and consciousness, knowing that you have received information from your own Higher Intelligence about that subject.

As you direct your thoughts to a person, notice the feelings that arise. If resistance arises, there is something not-clear with that person. Let it be not-clear for now, and withdraw your attention, returning to your own clear space, and your own personal clarity, to what is true for you.

Be honest with yourself, and identify any non-clarity you have with that person. If the basis for it is that you have decided what the other person should do, and your demands are not being met, release that decision, and acknowledge the other person's freedom. If the basis for the resistance is that demands have been placed on you, decide to not accept them, and acknowledge your own freedom. If the basis for the resistance is just that there are two different vibrations which bump into each other, and are by nature non-harmonious together, acknowledge that, and allow movement in different directions, for the sake of harmony for all.

If your consciousness is clear, and the resistance is something happening within the other person's consciousness, know that you are not responsible for what the other person chooses to think or feel. Send them love, and know that they can get through their own stuff, and that they will if and when they choose to. If you can help them, through some communication, in order to release misperceptions then do it, if you are inclined to. Otherwise, see them with compassion, understanding their perceptions, and knowing that there's nothing you can do about it unless they are open to your help. The love you send is unconditional, and is simply a wish for them that they find happiness their way.

By doing all of this, you can release the resistance in your own consciousness, the excess baggage you have been responsible for and which you have been carrying around. You are also recognizing that others are responsible for their baggage, and free to release it when they choose.

When your relationship with yourself is clearer, and lighter, your relationships with others will be, also. There will be a new basis for relating, with mutual acknowledgment, and much more freedom and love. There will be more and more positive experiences for you in all aspects of your life – and increased clarity on all levels.

Affirmations

I choose clarity.

Acceptance and love lead to clarity.

Today I choose to see the love.

Chapter 12

Be Here Now

Be who you really are in the moment of experience, the here and now. Do what you do consciously, with awareness. For example, eat only when you are really hungry, not just because it's time to eat. Eat what you really want now, not what you are habitually accustomed to eating, or what someone else thinks you should eat. If you want to be with people who are eating, but you're not hungry, just be with them without eating. Sleep when your body asks for it, not just when it's 'time to sleep.' It's about listening to your body, and living the moment of direct experience, rather than what your mind tells you.

Who you are is reflected in the constant NOW, the ever-present moment of experience. It is helpful during your day, to consciously return to NOW. Ask yourself:

What's happening now, and how do I feel about it?

What do I want to do now?

What is my life like now?

Am I putting off my dreams, or am I living them now?

This moment of life is important. How much of it am I experiencing now?

This is what my life is now – what is it that I'd really like to do with it?

Look at this page now. Notice the letters and their shapes, the size of the page, and the distance between letters and lines. Notice how clearly you see, whether or not you are wearing your eyeglasses. And now, keeping your eyes fixed on the letters and the page, think of what you had for dinner last night, what it tasted like, where you were, and whom you were with. Take a moment and do this now, while still watching this page. Go on, re-create last night in your mind.

Now, bring yourself back to the now and redirect all your attention to the letters on this page. You probably noticed that as your thoughts went to yesterday's dinner, today's page became blurred, but it returned to sharpness when your thoughts returned to now.

Vision exists only within the moment of experience, here and now. See things as they are now. Live in this moment, where fear and guilt do not exist. Fear lives in the future only. It is faith in a negative future. As you energize your fears by thinking about them and talking about them, you energize a future you really don't want, and by focusing on the negative future, you keep yourself from living in the present moment and enjoying what you do have.

You can decide instead to energize only a positive future by thinking about that, and then release it, and redirect your attention to the present moment, to what is happening around you now.

Guilt lives only in the past. It is faith in a negative past, where you believe you did something wrong, and the pre-occupation about that also keeps you from experiencing the now. Learn from the past, decide what you will do differently in the future, and then release the past. You have learned what you were supposed to from the experience in the evolution of your soul, on your path to clarity. Direct your attention to the present, and live it – now.

Trust heals fear.

Forgiveness heals guilt.

There are moments in time when we are experiencing something so important to us that we know we are in the right place, doing the right thing, with the right person or people. During these moments, there is a sense of perfection, and we see that all of the events leading up to these moments were perfect, and that they happened exactly as they were supposed to.

Perhaps you went shopping, and without knowing why, you bought something because it felt right in that moment to do that, although you had no reason to. Later in the day, you met someone you didn't expect to meet, and the reason for your impulse purchase became clear. What you bought was obviously meant for them – even though on a conscious level you had no idea you would be seeing them! Your intuition was working perfectly.

Or perhaps you missed an appointment, and because of that you met someone, and talked with them about something important to you. This talk resolved something for you. So, you had to miss the appointment in order to meet that person, so that you could learn about that book or that meeting. Then you discover it was no problem to have missed the appointment anyway. You see the perfection, and you know that at least for the events leading up to that perfect moment you did everything you were really supposed to, even though it didn't seem like it at the time.

When you experience a number of moments like that, you can see two models of the way the Universe is moving. In one model, there are accidents and coincidences, and things you did wrong. In the other model, everything is working perfectly, and you did everything you were really supposed to, in order to be happy. The end result was the real intention of your actions, for everyone's happiness.

Which model would you like to consider the real one, and which one is the illusion? When things happen that you don't understand, rather than feeling bad, you can remind yourself of the idea that it's all working perfectly, and some time in the future you'll see how it was all perfect. You can then release yourself to the present moment – the here and now – and live it, noticing the perfection more and more.

As this becomes a new habit, fear and guilt no longer make sense. You trust the Universe, and live in the now, with more happiness, and clearer vision. You are then able to experience more love. You notice the world is, after all, full of people motivated by love, and sometimes reacting to the perception that it isn't there. The misperception can be cleared through communication, and again, you learn to trust the present moment more and more.

Through all of these processes, tensions are released, and your vision becomes clearer and clearer.

Notice how your decision-making processes work. If, for example, there is a decision you will have to make next week, how much time will you spend between now and then thinking about it? If you do that, you will not be living in the here and now.

One moment you may decide, "I will do this." Then, you get another piece of information and you say, "No, I will do that." Then something else happens and you change your mind again. You can waste much of your now pre-deciding your decision, or you can instead say to yourself, "I'll decide to not decide until it's time to decide. At that time, I'll have all the information I need for the decision." You have then freed your present moment of experience, to be present within it.

When you live within the present moment, you may realize that it's not necessary to sacrifice the present moment for the future. How many times, when you're having a really good time, have you decided to stop because of what you have to do the next day? How many of the things you do today are things you don't enjoy for their own sake, but rather for the effects they may bring in the future?

When you live in the present moment, your actions are done because that's what you really want to do. You can then be totally present with what you are doing. You can be real, and not pretend to enjoy something you really don't like.

When you live in the present moment, you are not caught in the illusions of past and future. You are not led into situations by promises of how good it's going to be. You're able to focus your attention on the present, how it feels now, and what your instincts are saying about what is happening now.

Your instincts tell you what you need to know now, about what you are doing now. After all, your life is just a series of present moments of experience, just a sequence of 'NOW's.' You can learn to trust the present moment more and more, to live more and more in the now, where your vision is clearest.

Examine your average day, and notice how many of your experiences are investments in time for the future. How many people actually get to live that future, and how many continue to deny their todays for the tomorrows they may never experience? How many people live their lives as a dress rehearsal, preparing for Some Day When It Will All Be Perfect? The movie is rolling now. This is it.

Start living your life now, or when it's all over, your final thoughts will be a lot of "I wish I had..." thoughts. When I faced death the first time, that's what it was for me. I was shocked! What a sad way to end a life, thinking of all the things I could have done but didn't. I can assure you that it's much better to be able to say, "I'm glad I did..."

Since I've had several death experiences, I've met and spoken with other people who have also been across and back and we've compared experiences. One woman I spoke with was sure that when she got to the other side there was going to be a Being with a big book of her life, giving her good marks and bad marks, checks and crosses. I asked her what happened when she actually got there, and she told me it was, in fact, like that. She said there was a big book with checks and crosses, but the only crosses were for the things she hadn't done. In her case, as in so many others, self-denial was her only sin.

Acceptance can be used as a key to life in the present moment. Acceptance of yourself and your individuality, and acceptance of what is true for you. It can also be emotional acceptance of what is. Acceptance of other people's individuality also allows you to see them in the present – as they are – rather than how you would like to see them, different in some way. Release of past perceptions can be a conscious process, allowing you to see what is true now.

As you exist more in the now, your consciousness will be clearer, and so will your eyesight.

If you do find your perceptions not in the now – thinking of pasts and futures and not feeling good – you can use your eyesight to bring yourself back into the moment of experience, the here and now. Pick something to look at – it doesn't matter what it is. It can be a table, a carpet, your hand, a flower...whatever. Put all your attention onto it. Notice the colors, the texture, and just focus more and more of your attention on the visual field. Don't be concerned about clarity; just notice what you do see, until you notice all of your consciousness is involved with your visual experience in the Now.

Then you can look around in the present moment and notice what is going on around you. You may find colors are brighter and clearer, and in fact, your vision is a bit clearer. You have also released from your consciousness the not-good feelings of pasts and futures and can now keep your attention on something that feels good in the present.

Keep yourself present. With practice, this will become a new habit, and you will continue to notice the improved clarity of your vision.

Affirmations

I see clearly when I am here now.

Clarity exists here and now.

I see more clearly now.

Chapter 13

Bubble Reality

There is a story about a Zen master walking along a road and meeting a traveler going in the opposite direction. The traveler hailed the Zen master, and asked what life was like in the town he was headed toward, the one the Zen master had just left. The Zen master asked the traveler what life was like in the town the traveler had just come from. The traveler replied that people were irritable and mean, and not particularly honest. The Zen master told the traveler he was likely to find the same thing and the same kind of people in the town he was headed toward.

A bit further along the road, the Zen master met another traveler going in the opposite direction, and he had the same question as the previous traveler. When the Zen master asked this one what life was like in the town this traveler had just come from, the traveler replied that people had been open and friendly, always helpful and acting with integrity. The Zen master told this traveler he was likely to find the same thing and the same kind of people in the town he was headed toward.

Both travelers were headed for the same town, but a different field of energy – a different perceptual filter – surrounded each of them. Each was attracting a particular quality of experience determined by their particular energy field.

Each of us is surrounded by a bubble, which is the filter to our perceptions. All our perceptions must pass through this bubble, which filters and selects only the information we have decided is relevant to us at that time. The bubble is necessary, since we are surrounded with so much information coming in: what everyone is wearing, each person's face, all of the details of our environment, the number of leaves on a tree, the temperature, the dimensions of each cloud in the sky, all of the sounds we hear, and so on. If we had no selection process, we would experience chaos, as though we were watching a television set with all of the channels playing simultaneously.

It's like all of the information available in a computer. It's not all necessary or useful at one time, but as long as it's in the computer, we can access it when we need it. So, all of the information coming in doesn't need to register in our conscious awareness. It passes through the bubble unnoticed, yet is accessible when it's needed, either through conscious recall, or techniques such as hypnosis and regression.

If we imagine that each bubble is, for example, a particular color, we can say that someone is seeing the world through a red bubble, or a blue bubble, and so on.

Of course, through a red bubble, the world looks red, and through a blue bubble, the world looks blue. In actuality, the world may be neither red nor blue, but perhaps black and white. Imagine someone in a blue bubble and someone in a red bubble discussing the color of the world. Each would be certain they were right – and in fact, they would be right from their point of view, seen through their bubble. Each would be accurately reporting their perspective. We could say that they would both be right. We could also say that neither was right, in terms of the absolute reality that each was seeing through their respective filters. We could, however, say that each was accurately reporting their experience, and then we could get a sense of the bubble through which each was seeing.

We could say that each bubble is a product of that person's consciousness, and that the inside of each bubble is a mirror, so that people do not necessarily see the world the way it is, but rather they see it the way they are. Each person who is at the effect of their perceptions projects on to their view of the world their own intentions, and their own values.

When people judge others, they are in effect saying that if they were that person, they would be doing something wrong. They would be measuring the other person by their own standards, and perhaps, also measuring themselves by the standards of others. The view might be quite different when the other person's intentions, values, and reasons are known.

When others measure you by their standards, for example, deciding that you're wrong about something, they are projecting their intentions onto you. When you are able to communicate your intentions, often their judgments disappear. They are given the view from inside your bubble.

In any interaction it would be useful to have both views – the view from the inside looking out, and the view from the outside looking in. People who have been nearsighted have been more aware of the view from the inside looking out, and not much from the outside looking in. Whereas people who have been farsighted have been more aware of the view from the outside looking in than from the inside looking out. Both views are important, and having both views gives a more complete picture for intelligent decisions.

Perhaps you know people of whom you would say, "If only they followed their own advice." We could see, then, that they were seeing reflections of themselves projected onto those around them. Perhaps you, too, may have noticed yourself giving the same excellent advice to several people. Would that excellent advice be useful for you to follow, as well?

We could say that we attract to ourselves people to bring out from us information we need to hear ourselves. In a way, the world is full of people walking around talking to themselves – but only some of them are listening. After you realize this, you continue to talk to yourself, but now you can also listen. You can ask yourself whether this information coming from you is useful for you – and then follow your own advice. You could also see people who are giving you advice as talking to themselves, and giving themselves excellent advice. Only they would know, though, whether they were listening as well.

You can tell when your advice is meant for you if you are more interested in saying it than the other person is in hearing it. The words want to come out for you to hear. It works the other way, as well, when someone is more interested in giving you advice than you are in hearing it. It could be meant for them. When both people are interested in the communication, it flows. Otherwise, just notice your perceptions, and if you were to offer advice, notice what it would be. Inwardly, thank this other person for the favor they have done you on your path to clarity. You may then notice your view of that person change, since your perceptions of the past had served their purposes and disappeared, so you could now see that person in the present.

Being aware of your own bubble enables you to know yourself and what you are experiencing in your life. When you notice that you are projecting your own thoughts and feelings onto others, you can decide to take a fresh look. You can then go 'Through the Looking-glass,' and see other people's realities.

At levels of perception that most people experience, the mirroring process is not conscious, and so the people are at the effect of their perceptions. There is a level of perception at which these processes become conscious, and direct experiences, and that is at the level of the heart, seen through the bubble of unconditional love, of acceptance. With a direct view of others as yourself, there is compassion, understanding, and wisdom, and you find yourself talking to these people as though they were you, speaking with them in a way that you would like to be spoken to.

When you find yourself judging, you can be aware of it and use the awareness to raise the level of your perceptions to that of acceptance. The effect then is a release of tensions from your consciousness.

When you think of someone and feel resistance towards him or her, think of the quality of that person you feel the resistance about. What words would you use to describe that person? Ask yourself whether those words could be used to describe you, whether you can remember a time when you could have been described with those words, perhaps by someone who was not aware of the motives behind your actions and words .

Realize that this other person may have exactly the same motives, and you will sense a recognition and compassion for them. You will see them as yourself. It will be a new perception, and you could use that new perception as a basis for communication. Where before there was a wall between you, now there is an open door, a channel for communication. You could offer them the advice you would have appreciated getting. You could talk to them in the same way you would like to have been spoken to.

You can also recognize a person's characteristics without feeling resistance. The resistance tells you something about yourself. If you see the characteristic without resistance, without judging what the other person should do differently, you can decide what you need to do. For example, if someone is a thief, you can see it and do what is necessary to not have something stolen from you. You do not, however, need to be upset about their being a thief. You don't need to carry around resistance about that. They may, in fact, be a lovable thief, and perhaps even easier to love at a distance.

As you continue to remove resistance from your perceptions, you will be changing the nature of your bubble. You will see more and more that your consciousness has the means to answer all your questions, and give you all the guidance you need.

You will see more and more that you can be your own authority, your own guide, your own guru, your own Master, trusting more and more your own perceptions. You will more and more be able to own your clarity.

During the transformation process, you will be changing the nature of your bubble. This can be a gradual process over a period of time, or there can be a finite moment of change. When the process is gradual, there is the realization at one point that your vision is clearer than it used to be, and this gradual process continues until it stabilizes at clarity.

When the process of change happens in a particular moment, it can be experienced in one of two ways. There can be the experience of the old bubble suddenly 'popping,' sometimes with a rush of energy, exposing the new bubble. This may be experienced in much the same way as if waking from a dream, and suddenly seeing what is true in waking reality.

The second way the moment of change can be experienced is as if moving from one bubble to another, as if two bubbles – like soap bubbles – were touching each other and sharing a common membrane. Then, the point of consciousness (which is what you are) moves from the center of one bubble, through the membrane, into the second. Each bubble is a paradigm – a set of all things perceived, a reality, a certain way in which things make sense.

The movement is first experienced by the point of consciousness, as things no longer making sense in the old way. Of course, for things to make sense in a new way they must no longer make sense in the old way. In the narrow slice of time that the membrane represents, the individual might experience this as confusion in their perceptions, chaos, a lack of meaning. The individual must then not look backward at the way things used to make sense, but rather allow the meaninglessness, as movement goes through the membrane between the two bubbles. If you experience this, you can then know that it's just the curtain, the transition, and that its presence implies the process of rebirth into the new paradigm, the new bubble, the new reality.

A new meaning then emerges. Sense emerges from the chaos as movement continues into the new bubble. Attention is best maintained in the present, looking toward the future, watching the emerging process, the rebirth. The process becomes one of discovery and delight with the new paradigm, seeing how things are in fact different in a way that the individual recognizes as better.

Something else happens as well. You will discover that your bubble was not only a perceptual filter, but also a kind of selective magnet, attracting a certain kind of experience to you, and also a certain quality of people.

With the change in your bubble, the selectivity of the magnet changes as well, and you notice a different kind of experience being attracted to you, and a different quality of people. This is the direct result of the shift in your perceptions. Remember that your perceptions create your reality. As your perceptions change, your basic beliefs change as well and as you change your basic beliefs, your perceptions change accordingly.

In accord with these changes, events in the outer world change as well, and a totally different story unfolds around you. It's as though you have become a totally different character, in a totally different movie. Not only has the view from inside the bubble looking outward become different, but also the view from outside the bubble looking inward, and in fact, also the environment of the bubble. If the bubble was in a glass of beer, now it is in a glass of champagne, or what was flavored soda becomes sparkling water.

For you, the reader, these descriptions may seem a bit abstract at first, but when the process begins for you, you will recognize what is happening. As you re-read this chapter later, the words will connect more with your experience, and you will know that what is happening for you is what you have waited for and wanted. You can then watch your process of re-birth with a sense of stability – and clarity.

Affirmations

*I know what clarity is, and I experience it
more and more each day.*

Clarity is my natural state.

My vision is clearing now.

Chapter 14

The Human Directional System

Each of us is a consciousness on our individual journey to perfection. We exist simultaneously on different levels of experience that we call 'soul,' 'spirit,' and 'personality,' yet for most people, their awareness is present at only the level of personality. The other levels of consciousness are conceptualized or perceived as 'Higher Intelligence' by some, 'Holy Spirit' by others, and 'God' by still others.

Regardless of the name used for this other level of consciousness, it is available as a guide that we can use to lead us to fulfillment. While many perceive this guiding energy as something or someone outside themselves, it is actually an aspect of a deeper level of our own Being.

When you have a deep desire, or goal, all aspects of your Being – all levels – are in alignment relative to that goal. In the same way, we can say that when you make a decision with total dedication to that decision, all of your Being begins to move in the direction of its fulfillment. A flow is defined. Events in the outer world also move in accord with that decision. Higher Intelligence seems also to be in accord with that decision, helping you to achieve it.

Your movement through these events proceeds optimally when you are totally present in each moment and listening to your inner voice, your intuition, or instinct, which is, in effect, your communication link with Higher Intelligence. In other words, your direction comes from within, from the inside. In each moment, you can ask yourself, "What do I want to do now?"

As you move toward what you want to do in the Now, pay attention to two things: your feelings, and whether the direction taken is flowing or not. In other words, is there flow or resistance? Emotions which feel good flow. Emotions which do not feel good, we can call resistance. Events which have a tendency to happen are flowing. Events which have a tendency to not happen represent another kind of resistance – we can say there is resistance to their happening.

The flow and resistance of feelings is related to the flow and resistance of events. The flow that we are talking about here is toward the fulfillment of what had been defined as a deep desire. The idea is to remove the resistance, or not resist it, and follow the flow.

It's as though you're walking through a dream, aware of yourself as the character in the dream. It seems that the dream you are watching is a story not made up by you – but of course, what other consciousness but yours created the dream you are watching?

We give another name to the consciousness that seems to have made up the dream, and then define a relationship with that 'other' consciousness. However, that 'other' consciousness is just a deeper part of your own consciousness, a part we can call your Spirit, or Holy Spirit, if you wish, or God, or Higher Intelligence. Whatever you choose to call It, you and It are different parts of the same Being.

When you make a deep decision with all of your Being, there is an alignment of all levels of your consciousness. It's as though you have decided that the dream should change, and having done that, you watch the dream change, according to whatever you allow yourself to believe is possible. Or, we can say that you ask the dream to help you with the fulfillment of your goal. The effect is the same.

We can say that from the level of Spirit, Spirit is watching the personality in its perceptual bubble. Spirit knows the deep desires of that Being in the bubble, and what moves that Being towards things and away from things. Spirit then places thoughts, images, etc., into the bubble, for the personality to experience, and then there is a choice to move toward or away from those things.

We can say, for example, that Higher Intelligence sees an important meeting that can happen with someone if I leave my apartment in exactly four minutes, and walk east. If I'm paying attention that day, I'll have an impulse to leave, and take a walk heading east. I may not know exactly why I find myself walking in that direction, yet I will be watching for something to happen. When I meet that person on that walk, I'll recognize it as the reason for having had the impulse to leave the apartment at that time. It will be someone I have been looking forward to meeting. Then, I can be totally present with that person, knowing that it is a meeting that was 'supposed' to happen.

If I was not paying attention that day, I might not leave the apartment on impulse, and Higher Intelligence would have to find another way to move me toward that meeting. Since Higher Intelligence knows everything about me – for instance how much I love pizza – it drops the thought, 'Pizza,' into my bubble. I think of pizza and remember there is a pizzeria a few streets east of where I live, so I head in that direction exactly at the right moment (Higher Intelligence also knows exactly how long it takes for me to respond to certain things).

On the way to the pizzeria, I might notice that I'm not at all hungry, yet my legs are moving me purposefully in an easterly direction, apparently toward the pizzeria. Before I reach there, though, I meet someone I've been looking forward to meeting, and then I know the real reason for leaving the apartment – the meeting, and not the pizza. The pizza was the initial motivation, but the end result – the meeting – was the real original intention.

We can say that since everything is working perfectly, and things are happening exactly the way we really want them to – whether we are conscious of it or not – then the end result is always the real original intention. We can recognize our real intentions at deep levels of Being.

We can describe the process in another way. We can say that when you set a goal, the fulfillment of the goal exists, and you are moving toward it. The movement is defined as a tunnel that travels through time and space to the fulfillment of your goals, interacting with the space-time tunnels of others, which are leading them to the fulfillment of their goals. When there is an alignment of purposes, interactions are experienced which serve all Beings concerned.

Optimal travel through the tunnel is experienced through the center of the tunnel, when the Being is centered, and present, and doing what they want to do now, because it feels best to be doing that. If movement goes to the sides of this energy tunnel, there is resistance to the flow in the form of a tendency for things to not happen now, and also in the form of emotions that feel not-good, for example, emotional resistance. Pushing against the resistance creates more resistance, until the individual chooses to re-center him/herself, and moves in a direction in which things have a tendency to happen.

While the pushing may have been experienced as a desire having a tendency to not-happen, it was really just a function of the moment of experience, the fulfillment not happening now, at this time. Listen to your intuition, as it guides you through the eternal ever-present now.

Attachment impedes flow, and obscures the individual's perception of flow. When attached, the individual's consciousness is not in the here and now, where the flow is happening. Have desires, wishes, etc., without attachment to them, but rather with awareness of whether they have a tendency to happen now or not-now. Move with what wants to happen now, and away from what wants to not-happen now.

Throughout, be true to yourself. Do what you really want to do, and don't do what you really don't want to do. Express what you really would like, and also what you feel resistance towards. Trust the flow, and know that it's leading you to fulfillment. It's a friendly universe.

When you can say honestly: "I love where I am. I love who I'm with. I love what I'm doing," then you are on course, and only need to be present with your experience of the moment.

If you feel that you do not love where you are now, if there is resistance, then your guidance system is saying there is somewhere else you are supposed to be. You'll discover why when you are there.

If you are not able to say that you love whom you are with, if there is resistance being experienced being with them just now, your guidance system is saying that you and this other person – or persons – are vibrating at different frequencies and you need to either be with someone else vibrating at your frequency, or alone at this time. Remember, what we are talking about are always instructions for the present moment only.

If you do not love what you're doing, you're supposed to be doing something else. Do it, then, and trust your path.

After a while, a pattern will be evident to you, a pattern of events unfolding, and people moving, and you will see why things have happened the way they have. You'll see that everything is happening perfectly, exactly as it is supposed to, for everyone's benefit, although the reasons are not always evident until afterwards.

Each person is following their individual guidance system, traveling through their space-time tunnel, interacting with others traveling through their space-time tunnels. Each person is on their path to perfection, experiencing fulfillment of what has been their deep desires and goals. Each is doing what they can to find their place of harmony in the world.

Affirmations

I can notice clear vision today.

I can have clear vision today. I can see clearly today.

I love when I see clearly.

Chapter 15

Questions and Answers

Q. What food is good for improving eyesight?

A. Your body is constantly telling you what it needs and wants, and it knows what is best for you. Trust it, rather than some 'expert' who you have believed knows better what your body needs. The difficulty is that all the 'experts' are saying different things. One says you must not drink water with your meals, while another says you must drink a lot of water with meals. One says count calories and another says it's the carbohydrates rather than the calories that are important. One says you need these vitamins, another says they're useless. One says you must eat only live food, and another says we must have some meat. Who should you listen to?

Some people say eating meat is bad for your eyesight, and that if you become vegetarian, your eyesight will improve. Well, whatever you believe to be true, is true for you. If your body asks for vegetables, by all means give your body vegetables. It's interesting though to notice that vegetarians wear eyeglasses also, and that Eskimos as a race had perfect eyesight on a diet of whale and polar bear, and no vegetables, until they were introduced to competitive western society, with its 'modern' ideas. Then, some began to need eyeglasses.

Studies have shown how children offered a variety of foods are naturally drawn to what their bodies need. We have a mechanism – our appetite – that attracts us to the food we need. All we need to do is listen to our appetite without over-ruling it with what we think we should eat, or with habits that do not reflect our real appetite.

Do you eat when you are hungry, or when it's 'time to eat?' Do you eat to be sociable, to be with others who happen to be eating at that time? You can be with them without eating.

Listen to your body.

Rather than letting your mind decide what your body needs, listen to your body's communication mechanism, your appetite. Trust it and what it says, not only about what you should eat, but also how much. Stop eating when your appetite says your body has had enough and notice how good you feel when you do this.

When you are eating, pay attention to how you talk to yourself about what you are eating. Your body is listening. The words you use to describe your experience create your reality. Remind yourself that what you are eating is exactly what your body needs and is asking for at this time, and therefore you are getting the nutrients you need to improve your vision. Remind yourself how each act of eating results in your improved health, well-being, and clarity of vision. The way you talk to yourself about what you eat is at least as important as the food you put into your mouth. It's your mental diet, learning to trust more and more in your own perceptions and self-sufficiency.

You are your own best expert. You know best what you need. Remind yourself of that as much as you need to.

Q. Can sexual habits affect eyesight?

A. No, but hiding, suppressing, or not feeling okay about your sexuality in any way can have an adverse affect. Listen to your body and what it tells you. Let yourself be real, instead of feeling you must live up to an image that you have defined, or that you have allowed others to define. Just be who you really are, and feel what you really feel.

When you're hot, you're hot. When you're not, you're not.

Enjoy what you enjoy with others who enjoy the same thing, and don't measure yourself or your sexual preferences by other people's standards. Define your own way of being. Define your own morals and ethics that work for you and result in your happiness and harmony. You will find that there is, in fact, a universe of other Beings who share the same values.

Trust yourself, and have a good time with your life.

Q. Why do people in our society become farsighted at a certain age?

A. The reason so many people in our society develop farsightedness in their middle years is that our society encourages the development of the personality which is correlated with farsightedness. We are encouraged to believe that our natural tendency is to fall apart and grow useless as we get older. It is true for us only to the degree we believe it, and to the degree we allow it to be true for us. There are many individuals who do not develop farsightedness as they get older. None of us have to.

We are taught that it is more blessed to give than to receive, and that to think of your own needs is selfish or egoistic. This idea, carried to an extreme, results in the farsighted personality.

People over 50 who do not wear eyeglasses are more alive, and clearer in their consciousness about what is real for them.

It isn't necessary to accept the limiting belief that after a certain age, you will have to wear eyeglasses. If you have already accepted the idea, you can release it again as being true for others to the degree it is accepted by others, and describing what is true for them in their reality. You, though, can realize you have a choice, and then insist on re-clearing your vision.

Q. What are 'floaters,' and what can be done about them?

A. Floaters are tiny specks which appear to be floating in the person's field of vision. The personality associated with this seeing of spots in front of the eyes is one in which there is a compulsion to control. It may be a compulsion to control others, to control one's Self, or to control one's environment. When control is released, the spots disappear very quickly, often within minutes of the decision being made in the consciousness of the individual who had been affected.

Q. What do 'organic' vision problems represent?

A. When the effect of the vision problem is blindness, we can say the individual is keeping him or herself from seeing what they want (will eye) and/or what they feel (spirit eye). They have created a sense of separation from the world – isolation – with nothing to look forward to. If we look at what was happening in the individual's life at the time the symptom began, we will find there was a strong shock, and the individual may have responded to this by questioning their own goodness.

Thereafter, the individual did not let themselves see what they really wanted or felt, but rather edited their thoughts and feelings, perhaps with the idea it was not okay to want what they want, or to feel what they felt. Since wants and feelings are part of the Human Directional System that guides us toward fulfillment, the individual has nothing to look forward to. They do not anticipate fulfillment. With cataracts, this process happens slowly, over a period of time.

The nature of the organic difficulty gives insight into the details of the crisis that was experienced.

Glaucoma, for example, is a pressure in the eyes that is not being released. There are tiny ducts in the eyes which normally function to release excess pressure, and these have become blocked. The individual feels pressured and is seeing their world with a lot of pressure. Relaxation techniques do much to slowly release the pressure, allowing the individual a more relaxed view of their world. A visualization for those seriously interested in releasing this symptom is to imagine that these tiny ducts are slowly opening, a bit at a time, until normal functioning is restored. The visualization should be used in connection with deep relaxation techniques.

Detached retina happens in a person's life at the time of a separation from someone. A severed optic nerve, likewise, happens at a time when the individual experiences a shock brought about by separation.

When it is clear that something happening in the consciousness coincides with the onset of the organic problem, and the organic processes 'causing' the blindness followed as a result, it must be considered reasonable that another process in the consciousness resulting in a return to inner clarity can then be followed by other organic processes reversing the symptoms of blindness. This is in keeping with Dr. Bates' idea that all impaired vision is the result of stress, and that when the function of vision (as a process in the person's consciousness) is restored the organic causes can reverse themselves.

Retinitis Pigmentosa – In the eye there are blind spots caused by pigmentation on the retina. The substance melanin is associated with pigmentation, and also with the pineal gland, and the crown chakra, which in certain Eastern traditions represents perceptions of unity or separation. When this chakra or energy center is closed, the person experiences a sense of isolation. As with any healing, it is important to look at what was happening in the person's life at the time the symptom began, and in this case within the context of crown chakra issues – father, authority, and/or a sense of separation or isolation.

Q. What are the chakras, and what do they have to do with eyesight?

A. The chakras are energy centers within the body. The idea is that your consciousness fills your body, and when there is tension in a particular part of your consciousness, you feel it in a specific part of your body related to that part of your consciousness. It's as though everything you experience in your consciousness is divided into seven parts, each part ruled and regulated by a particular chakra. Each chakra interacts with the physical body through a particular endocrine gland, and a particular nerve group, or plexus.

Each of the senses is also related to a particular chakra. The sense of eyesight is related to the solar plexus chakra, which also governs our emotions and perceptions about power, control, and freedom. Therefore, we can say anyone with impaired vision is experiencing tension in their consciousness about these areas in their life. When the solar plexus chakra is clear, the individual experiences ease of being and clarity of vision.

The colour associated with this chakra is yellow. It's interesting to notice that, generally speaking, people see more clearly in sunlight. An excellent meditation if you are working on and improving your eyesight is to put the sun into your solar plexus and wear it there. Consider what it is like being the sun – always shining, effortlessly, with no need to defend or assert itself. It is a source of energy, and in a way, the source of all energy on this planet. Imagine being the sun.

With nearsightedness, in addition to the tension in the solar plexus there is also tension in the root chakra, which is located by the perineum. This chakra is related to our perceptions of security, survival, and trust. Nearsighted people have tension in this part of their consciousness and, in a way, do not feel safe. Their response is to withdraw inside and the effect of this is a sense of contraction. The parts of the body controlled by this chakra through the sacral plexus are the legs and elimination system, and also the sense of smell. The colour associated with this chakra is red.

Farsighted people also have tension in the throat chakra, which is related to expressing and receiving. On the physical level it is related not only to the throat, but also to the shoulders, arms, hands, and the sense of hearing. A farsighted person's response to a threatening world is to expand, and not let things in. There may be difficulty with receiving without guilt. Sky blue is the colour associated with this chakra.

With astigmatism, there may be tension in different chakras, depending on which ideas or parts of the consciousness are distorted. For other vision problems different chakras may be involved. With all vision problems, though, the solar plexus chakra is always involved.

When work is done on the chakras – which are aspects of consciousness – there is a change in the consciousness, and the person can then expect changes in their life. The process of healing implies transformation.

Following is a brief summary of the chakras as they relate to the different parts of your consciousness. Where there is tension in your consciousness in a particular chakra, and a resulting symptom, you can clear that part of your life, and watch the positive effect on the symptom.

Color	Chakra	Location	Consciousness	Sense
Violet	Crown	Top of head	Unity/Separation	Empathy
Indigo	Brow	Between Brows	Spiritual Awareness	E.S.P.
Blue	Throat	Base of Throat	Express/Receive	Hearing
Green	Heart	Center of chest	Relationships, Love	Touch
Yellow	Solar Plexus	Solar Plexus	Power, Control, Freedom	Vision
Orange	Abdominal	Abdomen	Food, Sex, Emotions	Taste
Red	Root	Perineum	Security, Trust, Home	Smell

The chakras are a vast subject, and to describe them in any detail, a book dedicated to that subject is necessary. Several have been written, including one by this author – *Anything Can Be Healed*, also published by Findhorn Press. For anyone already familiar with the chakras, the above information should be able to provide some helpful insights.

Q. What can you say about hereditary vision problems, such as color blindness?

A. The type of color blindness gives insight into the personality experiencing it and this can be explored by considering the chakras and their associated colors. For example, with red/green color blindness, the individual does not perceive the difference between red and green, which in the chakra system represents security and relationships, respectively.

When I told this to a color-blind man in Denmark, he asked, "Is there a difference?" He was in a vision improvement class I was leading, and he could see by the response of the other students that they perceived some difference between the two. He recognized he had been "losing himself" in his relationships, and that he no longer needed to do that. It was recognition of something at a very deep level, and immediately afterward, he was able to tell the difference between the color of a red geranium in the room, and its green leaves.

When we see the relationship between personality types and different kinds of physical problems, we must realize also that children tend to imitate parents, and if the parent's way of being predisposes them to a particular physical problem, and the children imitate that same way of being or the same philosophy, then the children will be predisposed to the same physical problem. The fact that in some cases the physical problem can be released shows us we are not limited by our genetic predisposition. By changing our consciousness, we can release any symptom.

I do not believe there exists any symptom from which someone, somewhere, somehow, has not been released. I believe that ultimately, anything can be healed.

Chapter 16

Conclusion

What I have done in this book is to record the ideas with which I have been working since 1975. These ideas, when presented to people interested in improving their vision, and used by them for that purpose, have resulted in improved vision for many.

Since we are working with a variable here – the consciousness of you the reader and what you bring to the process – no guarantee of results can be offered. It can only be stated that in the past, others have used these ideas successfully, and what one individual can do, any other individual can do. Therefore, we can say there is a potential for you to have the same results as others if you apply yourself in the same way, with the same degree of dedication.

The ideas in this book are tools and as such, they only work if you do.

If you have decided to apply yourself diligently and with a sense of dedication, you will discover for yourself the deep nature of your Being, and the unlimited potential contained within. You will be able to live from deeper and deeper parts of your Being, finally finding that place within you that exists beyond any symptoms.

In this book, the subject of improving eyesight has been used as a vehicle to offer ideas that can be applied to many other areas of your life. When you discover what you can do in the area of improving your vision, you will see how you can change any condition in your body, and any condition in your life. You will be able to live with a new sense of freedom and aliveness.

As you have seen, the process is not just one of improving the level of detail in the picture you see through your eyes. It is also a process of putting your life in order, getting it to be exactly the way you would like it to be, and living the rest of your life happily being yourself. It is available to you. It's up to you to go for it, and to be willing to see what Is.

At first, you will be able to create and maintain a clearer state of consciousness than before. You will know that when you insist on functioning from that space, it will just be a matter of time before your body catches up with the consciousness within, and reflects outward clarity, too.

It's very helpful during the process to stay in contact with other people who think positively, and who can provide encouragement and reinforcement. These can be people who work in the area of improving eyesight, healers, therapists, Silva Mind Control graduates, or others in the human potential movement. There are also some open-minded optometrists who are not threatened by the idea of improving eyesight, but rather who are truly dedicated to helping people's relationships with their eyes and their vision, and who are willing to consider some non-ordinary ideas which have had that result in the past, and which can be useful and helpful for the process of returning to clarity.

Discuss your successes with people who are positively predisposed to these ideas, so that your successes can encourage others, as the successes of others have encouraged you. And after you have had improvement that has been measured professionally, please let me know by writing to me through the publisher of this book. I love success stories.

Have a wonderful journey to clarity, exploring the consciousness of the most fascinating Being you know – your Self! Do it as a gift to your Self, as an expression of Self-love.

Here are the words to a song from an old album, *A Question Of Balance*, by The Moody Blues. These words seem appropriate to complete this work, and to leave one final idea resonating in your consciousness:

Just open your eyes
And realize
The way it's always been.

Just open your mind
And you will find
The way it's always been

Just open your heart
And that's a start.

Section IV

Exercises

Love Your Eyes

As with all exercises in this book, eyeglasses or contact lenses should not be worn.

The best time for this exercise is at the beginning of each day. It's very quick and very important to the relationship with your eyes. Although it may seem difficult at first – perhaps even foolish – the benefits will rapidly become evident.

Basic Exercise

Look in a mirror at your eyes.

Keeping your gaze on your eyes, say to them aloud:

I love you,
And I always will,
Always!

If your gaze did not remain on your eyes the entire time, the exercise must be repeated until done correctly.

If you are more adventurous, you may wish to do the Advanced version, which is called Love Your Self.

Advanced Version

Look in a mirror into your eyes, at the person whose eyes they are.

Looking directly into the eyes of the person you see, say to that person, aloud:

I love you,
And I always will,
Always!

If you did not look directly into the eyes the entire time, the exercise must be repeated.

After a while, you will notice that person saying these things to you, and you will be experiencing a new level of Being.

Note: The idea of both these exercises is to simply be able to say the words aloud while looking into your eyes. You may feel a lot of things as you say the words, "I love you," either to your eyes or to your Self. Let yourself feel whatever you feel.

Keep doing the exercise, and the relationship you have with your eyes and with your Self will continue to grow more and more loving. You will see the effects in your life, and in your clarity.

Exercise II

Do Nothing

When you are in charge of your own consciousness, you can decide to do something and remain 'on purpose,' insisting on doing that thing, maintaining single-mindedness of purpose.

If you choose, for example, to sit still for fifteen minutes each day – as an exercise in mental discipline and relaxation – and do nothing during that time, you should be able to do it. It may feel like wasted time, yet you may be assured it is not. It may be some of the most valuable time in your day. Isaac Newton may have thought he was involved in non-productive time sitting under the apple tree, yet it's where he discovered the principles of gravity!

Stress affects vision adversely. When we are under stress, we do not see clearly, both literally and figuratively. Relaxation enhances vision, and is the basis for many vision improvement techniques. Doing nothing encourages relaxation. If you feel too busy to sit and do nothing for fifteen minutes, you may need this exercise much more than you realize.

It is recommended that the exercise be done in a seated comfortable position, without moving.

- Close your eyes.
- Sit quietly for fifteen minutes, doing nothing.
- If it feels like there is something you must do, let it wait.
- If it feels like there is something you must think about, put it off until afterwards.
- For fifteen minutes, there are no decisions that need to be made, nothing to think about, nothing to read, nothing to listen to, nothing to do.

If thoughts come up, ignore them. If they seem to 'catch' you, recognize this, and replace them with an affirmation, like, "It's easier and easier to see clearly." Repeat the affirmation until your mind quiets again, and then return to doing nothing.

Insist on doing absolutely nothing. Relax into your sense of just being. Let yourself just be. Your mind will relax, the inner chatter will quit and the pushes and pulls will subside. Each time you do this you'll be able to be a bit clearer in your consciousness, and the cumulative effect will become noticeable in your consciousness during the exercise, and in your daily life.

You will be able to experience yourself as a point of consciousness, just Being.

After the fifteen minutes, open your eyes, and take a moment and see what your state of consciousness is like. Does it feel the same as when you started, or different in some way? If it is more relaxed (and of course, it will be) take a fresh look around you through new, more relaxed, eyes.

If it feels afterwards that you want to analyze your experience of this exercise, you can ask yourself the following questions:

- What were the temptations to do something else?
- Are they the same each time you do this exercise?
- For what reasons were you tempted to interrupt the exercise and 'come out of your space?'
- What are the things that seemed to stand between you and doing what you had decided is important for you? With mastery of

your own consciousness, you can decide which has the highest priority.

With practice, the exercise becomes easier and easier, and its benefits more and more apparent. Among other things, it develops single-mindedness, builds a pattern of success in working with your mind, enhances clarity of thought, and puts you in touch with your priorities, the order of importance that things have for you. Your Do Nothing sessions will become an oasis from which you'll be able to refresh your consciousness, reminding yourself what 'just being' is like for you, and you'll discover the joys and benefits of living from that space – with clarity!

Exercise III

Progressive Relaxation

This exercise may be done sitting or lying down. Many people find it easier to reach more relaxed levels of mind without falling asleep by doing it in a seated position.

The idea is to relax your body, one part at a time, by deliberately focusing on each part. You start with the toes, and slowly work upwards, mentally asking each part to let go and relax and then feeling it relax. Then follows a visualization and the use of some affirmations.

Make yourself comfortable.

Close your eyes.

Greet your toes *("Hello, toes!")*.

Tell your toes they can relax, and ask them to relax now. (Example: *"Toes, you can relax. Will you relax now?"*)

Feel your toes relax, and thank them.

Greet your feet, tell them they can relax, and ask them to relax now.

Feel your feet relax, and thank them.

Greet your ankles, and ask them to relax in the same way.

Feel your ankles relax, and thank them.

Repeat this process with calves and shins, knees, thighs, buttocks, lower back, abdomen, middle back, stomach, upper back, chest, fingers, hands, wrists, lower arms, upper arms, shoulders, neck, jaws, face, eyes, forehead, and scalp. By the time you reach your eyes, you will be easily able to feel the tensions there, and release them.

After reaching your scalp, create a picture of how it will be when you can again see clearly, and put yourself in the picture. Imagine yourself after your vision has cleared, using your eyes the way you enjoy using them when your vision is clear, seeing clearly in an easy and natural way, without eyeglasses or contact lenses.

Hold the image for ten seconds.

Then, imagine yourself in the office of your eye doctor, seeing clearly, waiting to see the look on his face when he discovers what you already know – that you can see clearly!

Then, imagine being examined, and seeing the eye chart clearly. Notice the look on your eye doctor's face – it's exactly as you imagined it would be.

Hear your eye doctor say, "I don't understand this. Perhaps we made a mistake with your last prescription, because it's definitely too strong for you now."

Thank your surprised eye doctor, and go out into the world to enjoy the new dimension your vision presents to you.

The more the scene is pictured and remembered, the more strongly the reality is created.

Say to yourself:

*"My eyes are relaxing **now**."*

*"My vision is improving **now**."*

"Each time I relax like this, my vision improves more."

*"I choose to see clearly, and my vision is clearing **now**. All that remains is for me to notice it, and I'm noticing it more and more."*

When you say the affirmations – the positive statements after the visualization – agree with them internally, and mean them as you say them. Decide that when you get up and open your eyes, you will be seeing more clearly. You may say the following or something like it:

"At the count of five I will snap my fingers and open my eyes, seeing and feeling better than before.

"One, two, coming back slowly and easily.

"Three. At the count of five I will snap my fingers and open my eyes, seeing and feeling better than before.

"Four, five! (Snap!) Eyes open, seeing and feeling better than before."

You may notice when the exercise is complete that your vision is just a bit clearer, even if only for a few moments.

The entire exercise will take at least ten to fifteen minutes, if done properly, and you can pace yourself accordingly. The more the process is done, the more improvement will be noticed. Encourage the perception that your vision is improving, even though it may feel in the beginning as if you are making it up. After a while, you will notice you can definitely see things you were not seeing before, and you will know the process is really working.

Variation

A variation of this exercise is to imagine that as each part of the body relaxes, it glows with white light. Imagine that you can see it, and feel it, and as each part of the body relaxes more, it glows more brightly. At the completion of the exercise, you will experience yourself centered, filled with white light, and surrounded by white light. It will soon be evident to you that being filled with and surrounded by White Light, and feeling centered in it, is not a state of consciousness that needs to be reserved for periods of meditation, but rather one from which you can function throughout your day, with greater effectiveness.

Remember that relaxation enhances vision. We're not just talking about relaxation techniques for fifteen minutes at a time. Those are just a vehicle for a more relaxed way of living, a more relaxed way of Being, a more relaxed way of seeing your life, feeling better about yourself, your values and real feelings – no matter what they are – and being the fullest expression of who you really are. When your inner and outer Beings are in alignment, you will be healthier and happier, and you will see even more clearly.

Exercise IV

Hatha Yoga Eye Exercises

This is a classic, very effective approach to vision improvement. It is very useful and beneficial when done in a relaxed state of mind, such as that achieved in *Exercise III, Progressive Relaxation*. With these exercises, the eye muscles are gently worked by moving the eyeballs (only as much as is comfortable) in different directions.

Between each set of movements, rest the eyes and mind by palming. Palming involves slightly cupping the palms and covering your closed eyes with them – without any pressure on the eyeballs – and visualizing the field of vision becoming blacker and blacker. It may help to imagine a little person with a paint roller painting the field of vision blacker and blacker. It has been found that people with normal vision are more easily able to visualize black, so the idea is to create the symptoms of normal vision. When a person has all of the symptoms of normal vision, that person sees normally!

It should be emphasized – rather than "stressed" – that during the eye movements, the point is not to see how far in each direction the eyes can move, but only how far they can move *comfortably*. The degree of movement will increase as tension is relieved in the eye muscles, over a period of time.

Begin by doing *Exercise III, Progressive Relaxation*, to create the relaxed state of mind optimal for these exercises.

After reaching your scalp, and before counting yourself back to normal waking reality, palm for one minute with your eyes closed, imagining blacker and blacker.

Remove the palms from over your eyes and open your eyes.

Without moving your head, move your eyes up and down five times.

Palm for one minute. Imagine blacker and blacker.

Remove the palms and open your eyes, without trying to focus.

Keeping the head still, move your eyes from side to side five times.

Palm for one minute. Imagine blacker and blacker.

Remove the palms and open your eyes.

Move your eyes diagonally in one direction five times.

Palm for one minute. Imagine blacker and blacker.

Remove the palms and open the eyes, not trying to focus.

Move your eyes diagonally in the other direction five times.

Palm for one minute. Imagine blacker and blacker.

Remove the palms and open your eyes.

Move your eyeballs in an arc up, left and right, five times.

Palm for one minute. Imagine blacker and blacker.

Remove the palms and open your eyes.

Move your eyeballs in an arc down, left and right, five times.

Palm for one minute. Imagine blacker and blacker.

Remove the palms and open your eyes.

Move your eyeballs in a circle five times.

Palm for one minute. Imagine blacker and blacker.

Remove the palms and open your eyes.

Move your eyeballs in a circle the other way, five times.

Palm for one minute. Imagine blacker and blacker.

Count yourself back as in *Exercise III, Progressive Relaxation,* or as in Exercise IV, with Positive Programming. and bring your attention back into the room.

Do this exercise once each day until the vision is clear.

As the Hatha Yoga exercises are done, tensions in the eye muscles and consciousness are gently released, and over a period of time, the eyeballs will have a natural tendency to resume their natural shape, and clarity will return. The relaxation techniques can also make your life easier and more enjoyable, and will contribute to the clarity of your vision on many levels.

Variation

Some people prefer a variation of the eye exercises in which the gaze is held on a fixed point on the wall, and the head is moved in different directions, up and down, side-to-side, etc. When done in this way, you also exercise the neck muscles, restoring flexibility to them, and releasing any tensions that had been stored there.

No matter which forms of eye exercises are done, they are always done in a relaxed state of mind.

Vision Balancing

This optional exercise is like tightrope walking for your eyes, but with no possibility of falling! It's excellent for getting both eyes to work together, and is particularly beneficial for people who experience one eye stronger than the other. It can be included into any level of improvement program, as the Spirit moves you.

Get a piece of string about two yards (meters) long and three colored ribbons (one of one color and two of another color). Tie a ribbon of one color in the center of the string, and tie ribbons of another color halfway between the first ribbon and each end of the string.

You will now have a piece of string with three colored ribbons tied on it, measuring one-fourth, one-half, and three-quarters of the length of string, thus:

```
---------------X---------------X---------------X---------------
```

Tie one end of the string to a doorknob – or closet pull, for example – and seat yourself comfortably in a chair at a distance equal to the length of the string. You need to be able to hold the string to the end of your nose so it will be taut between your nose and the other end.

When you close your right eye, the image in your left eye will be of the string stretching from the upper left part of your field of vision, to the lower right part.

When you close your left eye, the image in your right eye will be of the string stretching from the upper right part of your field of vision, to the lower left part.

With both eyes open, the two images will blend together You'll see one string going from the upper right to the lower left, and another string going from the upper left to the lower right. The two strings will appear to cross at some point.

If one image is stronger than the other, and one string is seen more distinctly than the other, you will be able to move your attention to the other eye until both strings are seen equally well. If there is some difficulty at first, it will be because you have not been accustomed to an equal balance between the two halves of your brain. This exercise stimulates communication between the two halves of your brain, as well as balancing your eyes. It may take some moments of orientation, but you can do it!

Moving the Cross Exercise

Notice where the two strings seem to cross. By moving your consciousness, you'll be able to determine where the two strings cross, and exercise your eyes and your consciousness at the same time.

1. Make the images cross at the center ribbon. Hold the image there for one minute.

2. Make the images cross at the nearer ribbon. Hold the image there for one minute.

3. Make the images cross at the center ribbon again. Hold the image there for one minute.

4. Make the images cross at the further ribbon. Hold the image there for one minute.

5. Make the images cross one more time at the center ribbon. Hold the image there for one minute.

This exercise does not take much time, so it will be easy to work it into your schedule. With practice this exercise will become easier and easier, and it will give you rapid positive feedback about the improvement of your vision.

Vision Affirmations

1. My vision is improving now.
2. I choose clarity.
3. I know what clarity is, and I experience it more and more each day.
4. I remember clarity, and I am returning to clarity.
5. I notice that I see more clearly every day.
6. I know I can see clearly now.
7. I know that my experiences lead me to clear vision.
8. I accept new ways of thinking and seeing which are clearer for me.
9. Acceptance and love lead to clarity.
10. I accept what I see, and I see more clearly.
11. It's easier and easier to see clearly.
12. I'm letting myself be real, and watching my vision clear.
13. It's more and more comfortable to be myself, and see clearly.
14. My mind is reaching out and bringing to my awareness any information I need to experience clear vision.
15. I can have clear vision today. I can see clearly today.
16. Every day, in every way, I'm getting better and better.
17. I see more clearly when I'm relaxed and centered.
18. I see clearly when I am here now.
19. Clarity exists here and now.
20. Clarity is my natural state.
21. Clarity is what is true for me.
22. I enjoy seeing clearly.
23. I see that everything is working perfectly.
24. I love when I see clearly.
25. Clarity is freedom, and being real.
26. I see more clearly now.
27. I see more clearly than I did before.
28. Today I choose to see the love.

29. When I do what I really want to do, something wonderful always happens.
30. I trust being real, and I see clearly.
31. I see clarity coming.
32. I can notice clear vision today.
33. As I clear my life, my vision clears.
34. My vision is clearing now.
35. I am free!
36. My vision continues to clear as I adjust to my new state of consciousness.
37. Instead of problems, I see solutions. I see the way things can work.
38. Clearing my vision is easier than I thought.
39. I know I can see clearly without eyeglasses.
40. I agree with these statements.
41. Affirmations always work!

Recommended Two-Month Program

Start each day with *Exercise I, Love Your Eyes*.

Each day, take some time to read one chapter in this book, as well as all the Affirmations. Practice Talking to Yourself (Chapter Nine).

While the times you choose for exercise periods are optional, the ideal times are early morning, or early evening, or mid-day – in that order.

One exercise period each day is good.

Two exercise periods each day is excellent.

Three exercise periods each day is *optimal.

*For the 'Optimal' program, daily entries in a 'Progress Journal' are excellent. Entries may be made at the end of each day, noting positive experiences related to the improvement.

As a guide, use the Program Chart that follows. After two months, review your degree of improvement. If the process is not yet complete, get weaker eyeglasses as appropriate, and repeat the process from Week 3. Continue until vision is satisfactorily clear, and eyeglasses are no longer necessary.

While the Progressive Relaxation and Hatha Yoga Eye Exercises are simple and easy to memorize, you may prefer to record them in your own voice on a cassette tape, with pleasant music or nature sounds in the background. Or you may prefer a professionally pre-pared vision improvement CD, which may be ordered from the publisher of this book (see back of book for details).

Two-month daily program chart

	GOOD	EXCELLENT	OPTIMAL
Week 1			
Start of Day:	Love Your Eyes (I) Read Affirmations	Love Your Eyes (I) Read Affirmations	Love Your Eyes (I) Read Affirmations
*Exercise Periods	1. Do Nothing (II)	1. Do Nothing (II) 2. Progressive Relaxation (III)	1. Do Nothing (II) 2. Progressive Relaxation (III) 3. Hatha Yoga Eye Exercises (IV)
During Day:	Talk to Yourself Read A Chapter	Talk to Yourself Read A Chapter	Talk to Yourself Read A Chapter
End of Day:			Read Affirmations Progress Journal
Week 2			
Start of Day:	Love Your Eyes (I) Read Affirmations	Love Your Eyes (I) Read Affirmations	Love Your Eyes (I) Read Affirmations
*Exercise Periods	1. Progressive Relaxation(III)	1. Do Nothing (II) 2. Eye Exercises(IV)	1. Do Nothing (II) 2. Progressive Relaxation (III) 3. Hatha Yoga Eye Exercises (IV)

During Day:	Talk to Yourself Read A Chapter	Talk to Yourself Read A Chapter	Talk to Yourself Read A Chapter
End of Day:			Read Affirmations Progress Journal

Week 3 to 8

Start of Day:	Love Your Eyes (I) Read Affirmations	Love Your Eyes (I) Read Affirmations	Love Your Eyes (I) Read Affirmations
***Exercise Periods**	1. Eye Exercises (IV)	1. Progressive Relaxation (III) 2. Positive Programming (III)	1. Do Nothing (II) 2. Progressive Relaxation (III) 3. Hatha Yoga Eye Exercises (IV)
During Day:	Talk to Yourself Read A Chapter	Talk to Yourself Read A Chapter	Talk to Yourself Read A Chapter
End of Day:			Read Affirmations Progress Journal

Week 9

Examine Eyes. If perfect, celebrate. Otherwise, congratulate yourself on progress so far, and repeat weeks 3 to 8.

Note: Vision Balancing (exercise V) is an optional exercise that can be included in any level of program, at any time.

How to Use the Eye Chart

The eye chart is not intended to be a test, but a barometer you can use to measure your progress, to see how much better you are seeing so far. You can place the chart on a wall or door where it may be seen from a distance of about ten feet (3 1/2 metres). From time to time, look at it to see how much improvement you notice so far.

You will probably memorize the eye chart, and this is good. As you memorize it you will be able to remember what the letters look like, and you will be able to imagine more and more that you can see further down the chart. And when you imagine you can see further down this eye chart, you will be able to see further down other eye charts, too. Vision is a process involving memory and imagination, and since you will be using these facilities you will be improving your vision. From time to time, it may be helpful for you to have a friend read the eye chart to you slowly, as you watch it. You may be astounded to find the letters jumping into clarity as they are read, letting you know that in reality, you can see, after all.

Your copy of the eye chart should be loose within the book; if this is missing please contact Findhorn Press and we will send you one.

Section V

Success Stories

Susanne Nissen – Copenhagen, Denmark

When I started working with the Vision Improvement Techniques I had the idea that not only might they help me clear my vision but I also might be led to a more satisfying way of life by applying them. I was on the lookout for something to make me feel better, but was not quite sure what that was. Of one thing I was certain, I knew I wanted to see clearly again. When I used the Progressive Relaxation with White Light, and the palming, I felt more relaxed and at ease. My vision did improve, slowly and gently at times, and at other times I would experience minutes, hours or even a whole day of total clarity.

My life style changed gradually. Before, my life had primarily been based on doing what other people wanted me to do, so that I would get their approval and maybe their love. Now I saw this did not work very well for me. External appreciation can come or go as the wind blows. I was not able to please everyone no matter what I did. Instead I slowly learned to reach inside for the love I had been longing for. The Love Your Eyes / Love Your Self Exercise helped me do this.

I saw how I had always had good intentions and this released any guilt I had felt. I then found it much easier to do what I really wanted to do and feel good about it, regardless of anyone else's opinion. In fact, I discovered that people often do approve of me, and if they don't, I no longer need their approval. With this new clear conscience people can no longer manipulate me, because I no longer allow it. I do what I want to do, and feel freer and lighter because of it. Love flows more freely and easily between other people and myself.

Another feeling which surfaced during the transformation process was fear. I had felt and then suppressed fear as best I could for most of my life. This suppression did not work; the fear was still there. In the beginning I tested various ways of dealing with it and had only some success. Then one day I decided that I might as well feel it totally, maybe then it would be released. I took a look at the seemingly different fears and found they were all somehow related to death or separation. I had to accept these are facts of life.

I had spent years looking for security outside myself and had rarely found it. Real, lasting security was not in my money, job, education, home or my relationships with other people. All these things I had invested my energy in offered me only a limited or temporary feeling of security. I saw how nothing in the world could ever offer me lasting security, so there was only one place left to look for it – inside!

I am still in the process of opening to that inner sense of security and already I feel much safer than I have in a very long time. I have discovered how everything is really just fine as it is and I am allowing myself to feel that, more and more. My world is increasingly mirroring my growing sense of security. Things which were chaotic before have now arranged themselves easily, in their normal order. I have bought my own apartment where I feel at home, free and comfortable, and where I can stay as long as I like. In the past, I had shared other people's apartments, and didn't really have a feeling of being free.

I am in a wonderful school now, and I always look forward to spending time with the enthusiastic teachers and students. My old university did not suit my personal needs. I also changed my job and my new job offers me more freedom, independence and satisfaction than ever before. My friendships are growing deeper and more respectful. I am able to trust people more easily than before, while still not depending on them. All these positive changes have taken place during the vision improvement process.

Today I can create with my consciousness whichever perception I desire, and the world reflects this perception in one way or another. The safer I feel inside, the more the world mirrors this safety. When I feel free inside, my world looks less limited. When my heart is filled with love, the people in my surroundings mirror this, and even plants, animals, the sky and the sea become love.

At times I have wondered about the deeper meaning of the vision impairment I had developed. It became evident to me how I had unconsciously chosen this experience in order to meet with this system of healing, and thus open my eyes to another dimension of reality, where things do not happen accidentally, but are related to cause and effect. For the first time I saw how the spiritual dimension was not just mere philosophy – it can indeed be felt and experienced.

Rarely do I experience fear and guilt any more, so I am able to be more present each moment. The more present I am in a situation, the clearer I see and the more joy I feel. I am still in this process of transformation. It is not yet complete. The changes in the prescriptions for my eyes are relatively small so far:

	Beginning of Vision Program	Now
left eye	- 1.5	- 1
right eye	- 1	- 0.75

With just these changes I see more clearly than I did before, and am also able to do without eyeglasses and contact lenses. I feel more relaxed in my body and as a 'side effect' of working with the Vision Program, the allergy to grass pollen I had suffered in my eyes every summer since I was seven years old has been healed. Thanks to the Vision Program I am able to totally enjoy nature and summer sun for the first time in 14 years!

Ziggy Moller – Copenhagen, Denmark

I first met Martin Brofman in October 1987 when I attended one of his healing intensives. One of the first things that Martin said to me during that course was, "I saw you wearing glasses. You don't have to, you know."

At that time I was a bit nearsighted (-0.75 in my left eye and -

1.00 in my right eye). This distortion, however, was enough to make it impossible for me to read subtitles on the television and at movies without my glasses. It was also impossible for me to read at a normal distance street names, the numbers on buses, and so on.

The possibility that I could get to see clearly without my glasses was a new one to me, but I decided to stay open to it. I had already worn my eyeglasses on a permanent basis for the last time and now only put them on if there was something I needed to read clearly. But the possibility of managing without them at all was certainly appealing.

After this first healing course with Martin, I knew a lot more about how my nearsightedness was connected to my feelings, my thoughts, and to my consciousness. The healing process had begun. Colors and shapes had already become more distinct and clear. It was as if my vision had been dusted off. I bought and read Martin's first book on vision improvement – actually I read it several times. I put the eye chart on the wall and used it for daily feedback on my vision improvement process. I also used it as a daily barometer indicating my inner balance, and from time to time there were very noticeable variations, which told me to look inside.

When I quit wearing my glasses I realized that wearing them had not just been a question of seeing more clearly, they had also had another function, that of keeping a distance between me and the world around me. I had kept myself from being in close and open contact with the world and the people in it. I remember how I would put on or take off my glasses in different situations according to how secure I felt. My glasses had become part of my facade, my mask.

The previous year I had been in psychotherapy, it had been a hard and heart-breaking process and I hadn't got far in dealing with my issues. Now I was in a personal transformation process that was so profound, simple, intense, and joyful. My issues were now being resolved through my self-healing process in a light, organic, and definitive way. The main thing for me was to begin to see myself as worthy of being loved, and to see how much love I had in my heart that I could begin to let flow freely.

I very clearly remember a major turning point. Standing by the window in my living room looking out at the world, there was a sudden shift in my consciousness and rather than seeing the world as hostile and dangerous, I suddenly saw it as friendly. My reality had changed and from that moment people were indeed friendly towards me. My process was also about being visible, so I got myself a new bright orange winter coat. It was not the kind of coat you could sneak around in, hoping to not be seen. Slowly but surely I began to feel at home wearing it.

Much has changed for me since my first course with Martin. Prior to then I had worked as a psychologist. Now I advertise myself as a psychologist and healer. That is what I have become, and I want to be visible in my new role. I have even exhibited and sold paintings that I had done for my own pleasure! The results of my work on my vision have stretched throughout my life. Before I could not see how love and freedom could go together. Now I have both. Fulfilling a promise to myself that with the proceeds from selling my first painting I would treat myself to a silver and diamond ring, I met and fell in love with a goldsmith!

Jytte Tranberg – Horsholm, Denmark

At age 22, my vision started to become blurry. I worked with needlework and embroidery, and was very dependent upon clear vision. An ophthalmologist told me I was farsighted and unfortunately would need glasses of +1 strength for my work. He told me it was very early to start with eyeglasses, as 'normally' people do not get farsighted before the age of 40 – 45 years.

Less than a year later my vision got generally dimmer, so I went back to the optician and moaned my distress. He shook his head and told me the glasses he had given me should last me for at least five years, with no problems. After much persuading he finally agreed to do another vision test – mainly to shut me up I think. This test proved that not only were stronger glasses necessary, but also I now needed to wear them all the time. Suddenly I had glasses sitting permanently on my nose – and that was very uncomfortable. I was far-sighted, but also had troubles with double vision at a distance.

At that time the first small, hard contact lenses had just showed up in Denmark, so I wanted to try them. Again much persuasion was necessary. I was told I would probably be crying for at least a month until my eyes got accustomed to having a foreign body directly on the cornea. It was true. I cried my courageous tears through seven different models of lenses until we finally found the right ones.

Over the years my lenses became stronger and stronger. When I was 40 years old my contact lenses were +2.75, and I still had my 'old-age glasses' with an additional correction of +1.5 for working and reading. At 50 years old, I needed a correction of +3.25 in my lenses, and +3 in my glasses for detailed work. A total correction of between +6 and +6.5.

At this time, I started to get interested in metaphysics. I read many books and was always buying new stacks to read from esoteric bookshops. Among these was a little book by Martin Brofman about restoring normal vision, but more than six months passed before I started to read it. It was after a visit to my optician that I began reading. He told me things were deteriorating and probably one day I would have to wear thick glasses – and that even then I could not count on completely clear vision. It was an awful shock. The thought of not being able to do the work I loved and living in permanent dimness was scary. I realized that something had to be done and finally was so extremely thankful to my optician for telling me this bad news – because it woke me up!

I dug out Martin Brofman's first little book, and followed the exercises (as in this book) faithfully. I worked with my eyes for 30 minutes every day for three weeks. Then I went back to the optician, told him about my exercises and how many carrots I had eaten, and asked him to give me a vision test. He inclined his head, smiled good humouredly and said, "My dear friend, I know carrots are wonderful, but unfortunately there is really nothing to do. Nothing can be done to improve your vision. Don't give yourself any illusions. Be happy that at least your vision has stabilized these last months."

Having just enrolled on a four-day intensive course with Martin Brofman, I looked at him and said, sure of myself, "We will see in a month's time."

I had understood that as long as I used my contact lenses my eyes would not get any chance to change. With the lenses in they could not relax and once again find their normal healthy form. So the first thing I did upon arrival at the course was to remove my lenses. I had four days ahead of me with no needlework, driving, cooking, or reading – I could manage without my lenses and glasses. I had decided that I wanted a brand new clear vision and was prepared to do whatever was necessary to achieve it. At dinnertime others would have to tell me what was on my plate, I was often not sure whether my clothes were inside out or not, and I gave up using my eyeliner – but these were all small prices to pay.

As the hours on the course passed my vision got clearer and clearer, colors became brighter and inside me a beautiful light was kindling. I started to understand why I didn't see clearly – what it was I didn't want to see in my life: It was ME. The more I dared see of myself, the better my vision became. On the last day of the intensive, I could see everything around me clearly. For the first time in 27 years I was able to drive home in my car without any contact lenses. It was incredible.

Not only had I gotten clearer vision, but an entirely new world had opened at my feet. At once I understood that acting in agreement with my feelings, instead of counteracting them, would put my psychic body as well as my physical body together in balance. I started to conceive how important it is to accept me as I AM, instead of trying to be how I imagine others think I ought to be. This eternal fear – if one is good enough, clever enough, strong enough, beautiful enough, loved enough – is a block to happiness. I also began to accept others as they ARE.

When back home from the intensive I tried to place a contact lens in my eye to see the difference. I could not do it – it was like putting a razor blade in my eye. My eyes had been totally transformed. Then I took my two pairs of glasses and threw them out. It was a really great moment. The following month I used some old glasses of strength +2 for working and reading, and then I went down to +1.5. At that time I went back to my optician and told him I had thrown out my lenses. He looked like an enormous question mark. "It's impossible," he said, "It's just impossible!"

My optican tested my eyes and the result was a correction of +.75 in both eyes. He was quite silent for a while. Then he told me yes this could happen, but it wouldn't last long. He went on to make me a fine drawing, explaining about liquids and pressure. I just listened. All of a sudden he gave up and said: "I surrender. It's a miracle, because it can't be done. How did you make it happen?" I told him I had changed my consciousness, so that my feelings and senses had become coordinated with the actions in my life. He enrolled himself on the next class.

One and a half years has passed and I still have a generally fine, clear, normal vision. I do still need glasses with strength of +1 and +1.5 for reading and more accurate work, but that is a whole lot less than the old +6! I have decided to look at the outstanding issues in my life, which have not yet been resolved. In two months time, I will throw my last glasses away. Then I shall start to give some wonderful healings, and help others on the road to clarity.

Lis Schroeder – Copenhagen, Denmark

A few years ago, I wore contact lenses. I had worn glasses and contact lenses for about 26 years. I was nearsighted.

| Then: | Right eye -4.00 | Left eye -4.25 |
| Now: | Right eye -2.00 | Left eye -2.50 |

In 1986 I heard about the possibility of improving one's eyesight. I could hardly imagine it could be possible, but I became curious, nonetheless. I had been doing therapy for some years at that time, as client and therapist, so I asked one of my therapist friends who knew about some eye exercises to do a session with me.

We never got to do the exercises, though. I spent a few minutes to tune-in to the session, listening to some music, and I suddenly made a tremendous shift in my consciousness. I found myself sitting on top of a pyramid, with a God-consciousness. I was able to move around exactly as I wanted to, and my field of vision was 360 degrees. I was experiencing deep peace and calmness. Watching the sunrise from the top of the pyramid a sound was being released from a deep part of me. I felt crystal clear, and I knew that I myself was a God, and that I had access to all wisdom in the Universe. Then I shifted again and experienced only light. I was the light. I was infinite.

As my awareness returned to the room it soon became clear that tensions had left my eye muscles. When I opened my eyes, things were so much clearer. However, I did not stop using my contact lenses. I was happy to have them and never had any trouble wearing them. Out of laziness I thought it would be nice, though, to not have to cleanse them every evening.

At the end of 1986 I participated in a four day Healing Intensive with Martin. By the end of the first day I decided to remove my contact lenses for the rest of the course. I felt insecure and blind as a mole, only able to recognize people when they appeared right next to me, and being totally unable to see what was on the blackboard.

On the fourth day, we exchanged healings and I asked for clearer eyesight. After the healing I could clearly see what was on the blackboard. I immediately went into a state of ecstasy. However, a part of me tried to deny the fact that I could see clearly. It just seemed too miraculous and hard to accept after 26 years with blurry eyesight. Because of my internal denials and doubts I was only able to stay in that clear state of consciousness with clear vision for a short time and was soon back to my old, well-known blurry reality again. A lot of things needed to be solved in my consciousness and my life.

From that day on I could no longer wear my contact lenses. Every time I tried, I immediately felt extremely stressed and tense and had to remove them again. Instead I went back to some old weaker glasses and only used them when necessary.

A short time after, I was robbed for the second time in my life. The first time had been many years before when someone stole my handbag with my glasses in it. This time, I was robbed of my purse containing all my identity cards. I saw the connection – somebody had been so kind as to rid me of all manifestations of my old identity as a result of what had happened inside me. On the physical level a lot of things around me broke, crashed, or just stopped functioning. An old reality and identity was cracking on all levels.

The process increased when I participated in Martin's Vision Workshop in the beginning of 1987. What was it that I had to look at? What was it that I had kept myself from seeing? And which techniques should I use to be able to stay in a clear state of consciousness resulting in stable clear eyesight? I started using all the techniques advised by Martin in this book, determined to get to the root of this. I made up my mind to be willing to do whatever was necessary to fulfill the process, to be honest and true with myself for my own well-being.

There was a lot to learn about me. About my fears and how because of them I had done my best to make myself invisible. About how I was not true to myself and had never really accepted myself. About how controlling I had been and how I believed it only possible to be in this world by making compromises.

I went back in time to find the source of my fears. As a child I had perceived the world and my home as a very dangerous place to be in. I had been so shocked when I realized that my body wasn't perfect – my left side was a bit thinner than my right side and I could never imagine being loved looking like that! That's when I started hiding. To top it all, my family (with all the best intentions) asserted that what I could see was hardly noticeable. They denied a fact that I could see very clearly myself and this was confusing. How could I trust them?

Mistrust started to spread. I deliberately began not doing things well, where before I had been good at most things. When I was a success I had attention on me, and I wanted to direct attention away from me, so nobody would see my 'fault.' My fear was not being accepted. Whenever I did express what I saw clearly, I was told: "You just don't say those things. You have to pretend to not see them." So, I did.

I felt a loss of freedom and cut off from others. This made me feel separated and unhappy and created an immense tension in me. I so wanted to feel united, and at one with myself. I really wanted direction and guidance, but could not accept what I was given as being true for me. It didn't feel good.

What I actually did was to disconnect myself from my Higher Self, and from being guided by my own intuition. This was my deepest fear. It was a feeling of being not real, of not really existing. I have had to learn that I can feel unity within myself always, and nothing outside of me need ever again be a cause for me to disconnect myself like that. I can stay in touch with my deepest being. I have learnt to trust my intuition, to accept and trust I'm my own authority, no matter what. I have learned that listening to my own guidance is the safest and most perfect thing there is.

I have worked on the physical level also with the eye exercises, but the effects showed best when I worked in my consciousness. Every time I changed something, released some bit of old reality, I experienced clearer eyesight. I also experienced greater happiness. I just felt better and better, which again positively accelerated the process. I experienced success.

As an effect of all these inner changes, my life started to change for the better. My home has changed and so has my job. What I now do for a living is being who I am – a healer. I also have a peaceful, harmonious, and loving relationship with my parents.

The experiences I attract are all more positive and pleasant than they were before. It is constantly confirmed to me that this world is a loving place to be in, and I am loved for who I am. My sense of freedom has increased and I no longer need to feel 'trapped' in situations, circumstances, and relationships. I have my freedom to change whatever I wish and no longer feel a victim. I create what happens to me. I am responsible for myself.

The most important thing has been my decision – on a very deep level – to go through with the process, no matter what. Regardless of how long it would take, or what would show up, I had a total commitment to go for the best.

My deep commitment resulted in an easy way to work with my vision. Things I needed to look at presented themselves perfectly, in the right time and order, when I was ready to cope and work with them. They still do.

My eyesight is still changing. At times, I experience it as normal, at times crystal-clear, and other times as blurry. When it is the latter I know to look within. My outer vision has only little importance for me today, other than as a barometer of how I am. I know it will eventually stay clear as a natural effect of my growing inner clarity.

Robert Collaud – Morges, Switzerland

I accept and love who I am

I love where I am. I love what I do. I love whom I am with.

Simply by living to the full the basic principle of Martin Brofman's work I have been healed of depression and, as a 'bonus', of nearsightedness.

I say simply because it required no effort, no therapy, no particular technique; I just allowed myself to be me. I eliminated all the old patterns and conditioning I had allowed education, religion and my life experience to impose on me.

In 1987 when I attended Martin's workshop, I was nearsighted. For six years I had been wearing eyeglasses to drive. During that time my nearsightedness had become more pronounced and my lenses too weak; I was thinking about changing them because I could no longer read road signs. However, nearsightedness was actually the least of my worries. Since adolescence I had been living in a state of depression and I had become expert in the art of developing so-called psychosomatic illnesses, some more serious than others.

Doctors, psychiatrists, and tranquilizers had been helping me to tolerate myself. A year before the workshop, I had sunk into such a deep depression that antidepressants had to be administered intravenously. Afterwards, because I found it unbearable that my desire to live depended on anti-depressants and sleeping pills, I started psychotherapy again, even though I was fully aware it was yet another form of dependency.

I had long since realized that no other person, nor any medicine, could heal me. I knew that my family, friends, and outside circumstances were not responsible for the state I was in. I knew that only I could find the solution – but where? Over the past ten years I had been seeking through different religions and philosophies, and had learned relaxation techniques through Sophrology, Alpha Training, and Silva Mind Control. These methods certainly helped me to keep my head above water, and also to resurface during those times when I sank back into depression. However, the constant feeling of malaise within myself, the sickness in my soul, the emptiness, was still there, and I could not find peace. Some essential element was missing.

Then I attended Martin Brofman's workshop. Never before had I heard anyone speak in this way, and yet it was as though nothing Martin said was new to me; as though each word was an echo of a knowledge buried deep inside me. It was like I had always known that all power, all solutions were within me; that nobody was responsible for me and I was responsible for no one; that the God I had been desperately searching for is within each and every one of us.

At last I had found the essential element: unconditional love. I understood that each one of us is unique and perfect, and that we have no other task but to recognize and live this perfection. Without love of oneself, giving and sacrifice are not really an expression of love, but merely a way of seeking the approval of others. And, above all, I understood that one could feel and express this love, without conditions, to every being.

I no longer needed medicines or eyeglasses.

I finally accepted myself. I understood that being different and having different aspirations was not a defect; that it wasn't necessary to conform to social standards and the wishes of others in order to be loved.

Very rapidly healing spread into all areas of my life. I accepted my dreams and my fantasies and they began to materialize. By acknowledging that everything was possible, everything became possible. I had longed to work in the field of data processing but did not believe I was capable. Six months later my dream became reality, and over a period of 18 months one by one my professional ambitions came true. In my private life, too, there were important changes. I left my home, and thereby conventional life as a couple. It wasn't easy at first because I was still limiting myself through fear of hurting my family and my friends. But little by little I understood how totally being myself and living in a state of inner harmony, I was in fact contributing to the personal fulfillment and well being of those I loved.

I also realized that the sensitivity I had wanted to eliminate was an integral part of my innermost being. Now, it is through this very sensitivity that I express my being as a healer and teacher.

Since Martin's workshop I have not worn eyeglasses. I decided to undergo an ophthalmological examination in November 1989 for the purpose of presenting evidence in this account:

Nearsightedness in	1981	R 0.5	L 0.5
	1987	deteriorated, not tested	
Examination in	1989	100% vision in each eye	

Today, I see depression as a desire to evolve that is being repressed due to fear of the unknown. Fear is precisely one of the factors common to people who are nearsighted. I see where I was, and now I see where I am. Clearly.

The White Light Vision Improvement CD

Meditations created and guided by Martin Brofman

1. White Light Vision Meditation 31:53
2. White Light Eye Exercises 39:20

These meditations will help you get in contact with the real you, and restore yourself to clarity on all levels.

The first meditation is a progressive White Light relaxation through the body. Stress affects eyesight adversely, while relaxation is known to have a beneficial effect. The affirmations and visualizations which are presented at alpha are all intended for the improvement of your eyesight and vision.

The second meditation with relaxing non-structured zither music by LaRaaJi is the same as the first, with the addition of eye exercises. These are designed to restore flexibility to the eye muscles, which are said to control not only the movement, but also the focus of your eyeballs.

Whatever you visualize repeatedly, you improve the probability of happening. Therefore, you can imagine what it will be like when your vision is clear again. Keep putting this picture of the future in your consciousness, and keep remembering the future as the means of creating it.

Published by FINDHORN PRESS • ISBN 1-84409-026-4
available from your local bookstore
or directly from www.findhornpress.com

About Martin Brofman

A pioneer in vision improvement, spiritual healing, and exploring the nature of the body/mind interface, MARTIN BROFMAN is the author of the revolutionary book *Anything Can Be Healed* – a manual for the Body Mirror System of Healing, which he developed through his research and experience while healing himself of terminal illness in 1975. He, with other healers he has trained, present these healing tools and his original vision improvement techniques worldwide. He has facilitated tens of thousands of individuals in their healings on all levels, including their eyesight. Martin is the founder of the Brofman Foundation for the Advancement of Healing.

www.healer.ch

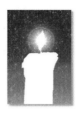

About Findhorn Press...

Findhorn Press was born in 1971 when the demand for the guidance of Eileen Caddy (one of the founders of the world famous Findhorn community) was so great that it was decided to publish it as a bound book: *God Spoke to Me* was launched and is still in print today! This was followed by many other books by Eileen Caddy, as well as several meditations tapes. Her latest title is the new (2002) expanded version of her autobiography, *Flight Into Freedom and Beyond*.

In 1994 Findhorn Press was purchased by Thierry and Karin Bogliolo, two long-term community members, and it has been run and developed as an independent publishing house since then. Its main office is still on the Findhorn campus but thanks to high speed internet connections several of its employees live in other parts of the world.

Findhorn Press has grown tremendously since it became independent, and publishes works by Diana Cooper, Martin Brofman, James F. Twyman, Marko Pogacnik, Darren Main, John Stowe, Jack Temple, David Lawson, Judy Hall and many others. While many of our authors are living or have lived in the Findhorn community, the others share the spiritual vision which is congruent with its core principles and practices.

Findhorn Press strives to bring healing and hope into our world. We seek to inspire and educate and inform our readers in every corner of the Earth – many of our books are published in several languages. Thank you for joining us on our journey into a positive and heart-centered future.

www.findhornpress.com

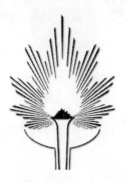

For further information about the Findhorn Foundation and the Findhorn Community, please contact:

Findhorn Foundation

The Visitors Centre
The Park, Findhorn IV36 3TZ, Scotland, UK
tel 01309 690311
enquiries@findhorn.org
www.findhorn.org

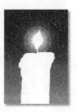

For a complete Findhorn Press catalogue, please contact:

Findhorn Press

305a The Park, Findhorn
Forres IV36 3TE
Scotland, UK
tel 01309 690582
fax 01309 690036
info@findhornpress.com
www.findhornpress.com